Handbook of Supportive Care in Oncology

Edited by

Ann Berger, MSN, MD

Bethesda, Maryland

CMP
United Business Media

Publishers of
ONCOLOGY
Oncology News International
Cancer Management: A Multidisciplinary Approach

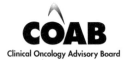

Clinical Oncology Advisory Board

Note to the reader
The information in this book has been carefully reviewed for accuracy of dosage and indications. Before prescribing any drug, however, the clinician should consult the manufacturer's current package labeling for accepted indications, absolute dosage recommendations, and other information pertinent to the safe and effective use of the product described. This is especially important when drugs are given in combination or as an adjunct to other forms of therapy. Furthermore, some of the medications described herein, as well as some of the indications mentioned, may not have been approved by the U.S. Food and Drug Administration at the time of publication. This possibility should be borne in mind before prescribing or recommending any drug or regimen.

Library of Congress Catalog Card Number 2005932887

ISBN Number 1891483374

Single copies of this book are available at $22.95 each. For information on obtaining additional copies, contact the publishers, CMP Healthcare Media, Oncology Publishing Group, 600 Community Drive, Manhasset, New York 11030. Telephone: (212) 600-3012, Fax: (212) 600-3050.

CMP
United Business Media

Publishers of
ONCOLOGY
Oncology News International
Cancer Management: A Multidisciplinary Approach

Contents

Contributing Authors

Ann Berger, MSN, MD
Bethesda, Maryland

Soenke Boettger, MD
Fellow
Department of Psychiatry & Behavioral Sciences
Memorial Sloan-Kettering Cancer Center
New York, New York

John Glaspy, MD
UCLA Medical Center
Los Angeles, California

Jimmie Holland, MD
Wayne E. Chapman Chair in Psychiatric Oncology
Attending Psychiatrist
Department of Psychiatry & Behavioral Sciences
Memorial Sloan-Kettering Cancer Center
New York, New York

Joyson Karakunnel, MD
Boyds, Maryland

Nicole M. Kuderer, MD
Postdoctoral Research Fellow
James P. Wilmot Cancer Center
University of Rochester School of Medicine and Dentistry
Rochester, New York

Gary H. Lyman, MD, MPH, FRCP (Edin)
Professor of Medicine and Oncology
Director of Health Services and Outcomes Research
James P. Wilmot Cancer Center
University of Rochester School of Medicine and Dentistry
Rochester, New York

Apurva A. Modi, MD
University of Texas Medical School at Houston
Houston, Texas

Douglas E. Peterson, DMD, PhD
Professor
Department of Oral Health and Diagnostic Sciences
School of Dental Medicine
Chair, Head & Neck/Oral Oncology Program
Neag Comprehensive Cancer Center
University of Connecticut Health Center
Farmington, Connecticut

Diane C. St. Germain, RN, MS, CRNP
Arlington, Virginia

Wendy L. Wiser, DO
Bethesda, Maryland

Preface

Ann Berger, MSN, MD

Great strides have been made in the treatment of the preponderance of cancers in recent decades, to the extent that virtually 50% of persons who develop cancer can be cured. Whether a cancer can be cured—or whether one can hope only for limited remission—what the patient feels most acutely are the physical and mental symptoms associated with the cancer, rather than the symptoms of the cancer itself.

Now, as has always been the case, the cancer patient is acutely aware—and acutely fears—those symptoms that we now consider under the rubric of supportive care. Supportive, yes, but lesser? Not to the patient! Fatigue and anemia, neutropenia, pain, nausea, constipation, oral mucositis, and—all too frequently (though understandably)—anxiety and depression are experienced, and if not experienced, feared, and these fears not only complicate treatment, but also have a detrimental effect on the quality of life of the patient and the patient's family.

Comprehensive texts on cancer have existed since the 1970s, and comprehensive texts on supportive and palliative care of the cancer patient have existed since the late 1990s. In addition to several splendid comprehensive texts (that can run well over 1,000 pages!), we have felt the need for a short, sharply focused handbook that enables the healthcare professional to quickly access the information needed most immediately at the bedside. The following pages have been written with that objective in mind.

As the treatment of cancer and the supportive care of the patient have become more complex, so have the responsibilities of healthcare professionals. As a consequence, we have solicited contributions in these pages from men and women who represent a range of professional concerns—

physicians, nurses, psychiatrists, and experts in public health and dentistry. Despite differences in professional training and perspective, and despite immersion in teaching and research, they have one thing in common—they focus on supportive care. They actively treat patients.

Anemia and Fatigue

John Glaspy, MD

Fatigue is common in patients with cancer, particularly in those who are receiving chemotherapy, and frequently represents the symptom that is most limiting to quality of life (1–3). Clearly, the increase in fatigue reported by cancer patients is multifactorial, with the following all playing a role:

- ❖ Inflammatory cytokines
- ❖ Sleep disturbances
- ❖ Depression
- ❖ Malnutrition
- ❖ Hormone withdrawal (menopause and/or antiestrogen therapy in women, chemical castration in men)
- ❖ Pain and pain medications
- ❖ Systemic effects of chemotherapy
- ❖ Liver, heart, and kidney dysfunction

One of the most important advances in supportive care since 1995 was the recognition that a significant proportion of the fatigue experienced by cancer patients was due to anemia, including mild and moderate degrees of anemia that had previously been considered to be asymptomatic. The correlation coefficients for fatigue and hemoglobin levels suggest that 15%–25% of variations in energy scores reported by cancer patients are explained by variations in hemoglobin levels (4). It is now well recognized that successful treatment of anemia in cancer patients is associated with improvements in energy levels and productivity (5–18). Hence, in approaching the fatigued cancer patient, it is reasonable to first obtain a hemoglobin level and address anemia, if present.

Treatment of Anemia in the Cancer Patient

Anemia is very common in cancer patients. Nutritional anemia, including iron deficiency (especially with tumors of the gastrointestinal tract) and vitamin B_{12} or folic acid deficiency, is not uncommon in patients with cancer and should obviously be treated with replacement of the appropriate nutrient. Hemolysis is less common, usually occurring in patients with lymphoid malignancies due to the disease itself or as a side effect of drugs such as fludarabine, and should be managed by removing any inciting drug or treating the underlying disease, adding corticosteroids, and considering treatment with agents such as anti-CD20 monoclonal antibody [rituximab (Rituxan®, Genentech)]. The majority of anemic cancer patients are found to have no nutritional deficiency or hemolysis; for these patients, the anemia is due to the anemia of chronic disease [cytokine-mediated suppression of endogenous erythropoietin production (19), resistance of the marrow to the effects of erythropoietin and the inability to absorb iron or access storage iron pools (20–22)] and the myelosuppressive effects of chemotherapy. The etiology of anemia in cancer patients is summarized in Figure 1.

Until the 1990s, the only modality available for the treatment of non-nutritional, nonhemolytic anemia in the cancer patient was red blood cell transfusions, with all the attendant risks and implications for the blood supply. The use of transfusions was and remains limited to the treatment of severe anemia (hemoglobin level <8 g/dL) or to situations in which the anemia is life threatening owing to comorbid cardiovascular disease, meaning that more moderate degrees of anemia, until relatively recently, went untreated. The development of technologies for cloning and producing recombinant human proteins has made the administration of erythropoiesis-stimulating proteins (ESPs) possible. ESPs act on the erythropoietin receptor (EPO-R) to promote survival and proliferation of red blood cell precursors in the bone marrow, increasing red blood cell production and hemoglobin levels.

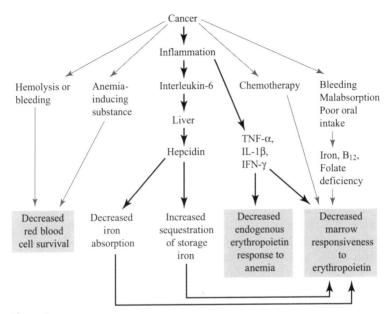

Figure 1
The etiology of anemia in cancer patients. B_{12}, vitamin B_{12}; IFN-γ, interferon γ; IL-1β, interleukin-1β; TFN-α, tumor necrosis factor-α.

Two ESPs are currently available in the United States for the treatment of anemia in cancer patients undergoing chemotherapy: epoetin alfa (Procrit®, Ortho Biotech) and darbepoetin alfa (Aranesp®, Amgen). Both of these agents have been shown to decrease transfusion requirements and, more important, to decrease fatigue and increase energy level and overall quality of life in patients with cancer who are receiving chemotherapy. In the United States, epoetin alfa is typically administered at a starting dose of 40,000 U/week by subcutaneous injection; darbepoetin alfa is most often administered at a starting dose of 200 mcg subcutaneously every 2 weeks, although, because of its longer half-life and the frequency of every-3-week chemotherapy regimens, darbepoetin alfa is sometimes administered every three weeks at a starting dose of 300 mcg. In Europe, there is a third ESP on the market, epoetin beta (NeoRecormon®, Roche), and the dosing of all of the ESPs are somewhat different. There is no definitive evidence that one ESP is more effective than another when applied to the treatment of anemia in cancer patients, and, in this chapter, they are in general considered together.

Who Should Be Treated with Erythropoiesis-Stimulating Proteins and When Should Treatment Begin?

It is clear from the available data that nonmyeloid cancer patients who are not receiving chemotherapy are frequently anemic, are at risk for red blood cell transfusions, and respond to ESP therapy, if anything, better than patients who are receiving chemotherapy (23–25). Because of differences in how the two treatment populations were treated in the pivotal randomized clinical trials of epoetin alfa (patients receiving chemotherapy remained on study for 12 weeks; patients not receiving chemotherapy remained on study for only 8 weeks), the observed decrease in transfusions in the latter group was not statistically significant. This has resulted in a situation in which ESP therapy clearly benefits patients with chemotherapy-induced anemia (CIA) and those with cancer who are not receiving chemotherapy (anemia of cancer, or AOC), but regulatory authorities in the United States and Europe have only registered ESPs for the treatment of patients with CIA. Coverage for any ESP treatment of AOC varies by payer and, for Medicare, by region, with coverage in approximately 60% of regions in 2005. It is important that the reader determine coverage policies for each patient, especially those with AOC. Because it is clear that the patients benefit and there is no rationale for treating them differently, this chapter includes AOC patients in the discussion of treatment of anemia in cancer patients. The safety and efficacy of ESPs in the treatment of patients with myeloid malignancies have not been established, and routine treatment of these patients with ESPs outside the setting of a clinical trial is not advised.

The only two benefits that have been shown to be associated with ESP therapy in cancer are a decrease in transfusion risk and an improvement in fatigue. Therefore, it is logical to focus therapy on patients who have fatigue or who are at risk for the development of anemia severe enough to warrant red blood cell transfusions. Initially, this led to ESP treatment guidelines that endorsed withholding treatment in the majority of patients until the hemoglobin level fell below 10 g/dL, when, it was thought, the benefits of treatment would be most clear and the cost of treatment was minimized (26–30). However, ESPs do not work immediately; depending on how low the hemoglobin level at initiation and, therefore, how great the magnitude of the desired hemoglobin gain, the median time to response is 6–10 weeks. In randomized controlled trials of ESPs, there is no difference between the placebo and ESP groups in transfusion risk for the first 4 weeks of therapy. A recent meta-analysis of randomized trials of ESPs concluded that the risk of transfusion is reduced by approximately 50% when ESPs are started early (hemoglobin, 10.5 g/dL or higher) rather than late (hemoglobin, 10 g/dL or less) (31).

The relationship between the hemoglobin level and the degree of fatigue is not a linear one. In a statistic modeling analysis of a large database of patients with CIA treated with epoetin alfa, it was found that the incremental gain in energy or quality of life from a 1-g increase in hemoglobin level was greatest for the intervals from 10 to 11 g/dL and from 11 to 12 g/dL (32). The modeled relationship is shown graphically in Figure 2. This observation has implications for the optimal approach to managing fatigue in anemic cancer patients. If the steep portion of the hemoglobin/quality-of-life relationship is in the range of 10–12 g/dL of hemoglobin, and, if there is a significant delay between the initiation of ESPs and an increase in hemoglobin, it makes sense to structure a treatment paradigm aimed at maintaining hemoglobin levels within the range of 11–13 g/dL for as much of the treatment course as possible. Earlier initiation of ESP therapy, in addition to further reducing transfusion risks, should be associated with substantially less fatigue and lost productivity for cancer patients. The rationale for early initiation of treatment is shown in Figure 3 (33). It should be noted that decreased transfusions and increased time within the hemoglobin range associated with reduced fatigue are benefits of ESPs, and, hence, this early initiation may be associated with increased cost benefit, rather than decreased cost benefit as was initially assumed. Clearly, more patients would be treated, increasing costs, and the impact of early initiation on cost benefit requires careful study. More recently developed guidelines for ESPs in cancer patients have recognized that early initiation is a defensible therapeutic option (34,35).

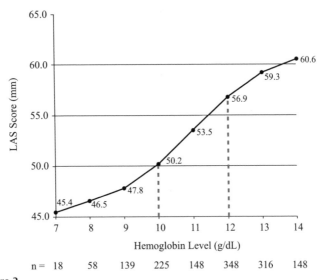

Figure 2
Hemoglobin levels in fatigue. LAS, linear analog scale.

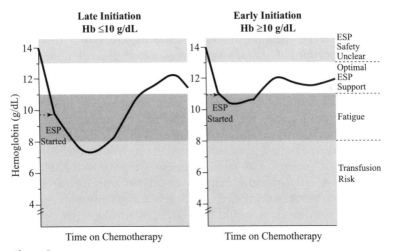

Figure 3
Iron-restricted erythropoiesis. ESP, erythropoiesis-stimulating protein; Hb, hemoglobin.

In some regions, early initiation of ESPs is covered by Medicare; in other regions, coverage is restricted to patients with hemoglobin levels <10 g/dL. If coverage is available, the current data support the initiation of erythropoietic agents in cancer patients with fatigue if the hemoglobin level is <12 g/dL. For cancer patients without fatigue, it is reasonable to initiate therapy when the hemoglobin level falls below 11 g/dL, particularly in the setting of CIA, in which further decreases in the hemoglobin level are anticipated.

How Should Patients Be Treated for Anemia?

Patients with severe anemia (hemoglobin levels <8 g/dL) should be considered for red blood cell transfusions, particularly if they are experiencing cardiovascular symptoms. For patients who have more moderate grades of anemia, ESP treatment should begin when fatigue develops or the hemoglobin level falls below 10.5–11.0 g/dL. In the United States, the options include epoetin alfa, 40,000 U subcutaneously weekly, and darbepoetin alfa, 200 mcg every 2 weeks or 300 mcg every 3 weeks subcutaneously. Both drugs can be administered intravenously, although this may be associated with less favorable pharmacokinetics, and there are less data to support this approach.

Adjusting Doses

A reasonable target hemoglobin concentration is 12 g/dL. Because hemoglobin levels fluctuate throughout the chemotherapy cycle, a reasonable and usually achievable goal of therapy is to maintain hemoglobin levels >11 g/dL and <13 g/dL. If a patient responds to therapy and hemoglobin levels are in this range and rising, ESP doses can be reduced or interdose intervals increased to maintain the hemoglobin level in range. If the hemoglobin level exceeds 13 g/dL, ESP treatment should be withheld until the level is <13 g/dL and then restarted at a dose and frequency that delivers one-half the previous dose over time. If the hemoglobin level rises at a rate that exceeds 2 g/dL in any 2-week period, a 50% reduction in dose or a doubling of the interdose interval is recommended (see Safety of Erythropoiesis-Stimulating Proteins for Cancer Patients, later).

A significant proportion of patients who are treated with ESPs for CIA, and less so for AOC, do not have a significant increase in hemoglobin level after 4–6 weeks. If the patient's hemoglobin level is still beneath the target range and a 1-g/dL increase in hemoglobin concentration is not observed within 4–6 weeks, a 50% increase in ESP dose is currently recommended, although there are no randomized trials confirming the benefits of this approach and it has substantial cost implications. Because the response to a given ESP dose can take as long as 10 weeks to become evident, the observation of hemoglobin increases in some patients for whom the dose is increased after 4–6 weeks does not definitively establish the benefit of the increased dose. Recent data strongly suggest that another better-documented option for the hyporesponsive patient is a therapeutic trial of parenteral iron.

Treatment with Iron

There are two ways in which patients with cancer who are being treated with ESPs can develop iron-restricted erythropoiesis, thereby limiting their responsiveness to therapy (see Figure 1):

❖ First, patients may have marginal iron reserves due to blood loss and/or decreased oral intake.

❖ Second, patients with adequate iron reserves can develop iron-restricted erythropoiesis owing to inability to access storage iron rapidly enough to optimally respond, a process termed *functional iron deficiency* (FID).

For dialysis patients or autologous blood donors undergoing ESP therapy, FID is a well-recognized and frequently encountered problem, and treatment with parenteral iron is shown to increase the response to ESPs. Because of the decreased iron absorption and accessibility of storage iron associated with the hepcidin produced by patients with chronic illnesses, such as cancer (36), it is likely that FID is, if anything, more common in cancer patients undergoing ESP therapy. Although the use of parenteral iron to enhance ESP response is currently applied least frequently in oncology, it, paradoxically, may be the setting in which it is most likely to improve ESP response.

In 2004, randomized clinical trials demonstrated that substantially greater increases in hemoglobin levels are observed in ESP-treated patients with CIA who are also treated with parenteral iron dextran (37) or ferric gluconate (38) than in those treated with oral iron or no iron. Of interest in the iron dextran trial, patients treated with a single intravenous infusion of the total calculated required dose of dextran [0.0442 (desired hemoglobin – observed hemoglobin) × lean body weight in kg + (0.26 × lean body weight)] experienced a benefit in terms of enhanced ESP response equal to weekly parenteral dextran therapy with 100 mg/week. The total dose infusion approach is attractive from the standpoint of cost and convenience, because each patient need only be treated once. However, some clinicians have concerns about the rare allergic reaction that has been reported in patients receiving iron dextran but not the newer iron salt preparations. An alternative is to administer ferric gluconate, 125 mg (two 62.5-mg vials). Given the current data, parenteral iron, and not ESP dose escalation, is the most promising approach to enhancing ESP response. The parenteral iron agents are summarized in Table 1.

Table 1.   Parenteral Iron Agents

Brand Name, Manufacturer	Generic Name	Dose for Anemia of Cancer	Comments
Infed®, Watson	Iron dextran	Either total dose infusion (see chart in PDR or equation in text) once or 100 mg weekly; no faster than 50 mg/min IV	Risk of hypersensitivity reactions; 0.5-mL test dose recommended Arthralgias more common with total dose infusion, decreased with methylprednisolone
Ferrlecit®, Watson	Ferric gluconate	125 mg (two vials) weekly for eight treatments	Arthralgias and generalized malaise more common if higher doses are attempted
Venofer®, American Regent	Iron sucrose	No randomized trials available for anemia of cancer	—

PDR, *Physicians' Desk Reference.*

The major challenge is in selecting patients for whom parenteral iron therapy is appropriate. The conventional measures of iron (iron, binding capacity, transferrin saturation, and ferritin) are adequate measures of iron stores in healthy subjects and patients who do not have chronic inflammatory illness. For subjects, including cancer patients, with the anemia of chronic illness, these measures are much less reliable. In this setting, ferritin is often elevated and iron, iron binding capacity, and transferrin saturation are often decreased by the illness, irrespective of iron stores. Moreover, even an accurate assessment of iron stores does not speak to the issue of FID, which by definition occurs in the presence of what should be an adequate iron supply in storage iron but is caused by an overwhelming demand on the part of ESP-stimulated erythron. What is needed are sensitive and specific markers of recent and ongoing iron-restricted erythropoiesis. Circulating soluble transferrin receptor levels are not confounded by the perturbations of chronic disease, but these levels are effected by chemotherapy, limiting their potential usefulness in oncology. Two parameters, percent hypochromic red cells and reticulocyte hemoglobin content, are probably the best markers of recent and ongoing iron-restricted erythropoiesis, respectively (39). When the percent hypochromic red cells exceeds 10, the clinician can conclude that access to iron has been limiting ESP response over the preceding 2 weeks. When the reticulocyte hemoglobin content is <29 pg, one can conclude that iron-restricted erythropoiesis is ongoing. Both parameters are relatively straightforward to measure in blood count autoanalyzers but, unfortunately, not yet broadly available in the United States. For centers at which these parameters are not available, a common sense approach is to administer parenteral iron from the beginning of ESP treatment to patients with transferrin saturation levels of <25% and to any patient who is or becomes hyporesponsive to ESPs during the course of therapy.

A proposed treatment algorithm for the treatment of anemia in cancer patients is presented in Figure 4.

Safety of Erythropoiesis-Stimulating Proteins for Cancer Patients

There are two safety issues that have been raised with respect to the use of ESPs in cancer patients: the potential to accelerate tumor pro-

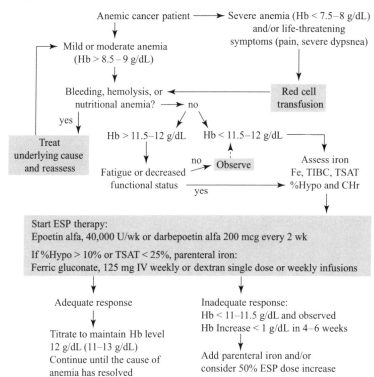

Figure 4

Algorithm for the treatment of anemia. CHr, reticulocyte hemoglobin content; ESP, erythropoiesis-stimulating protein; Fe, iron; Hb, hemoglobin; %Hypo, percent hypochromic red cells; TIBC, total iron-binding capacity; TSAT, transferrin saturation.

gression and an increased risk of thrombosis. Concerns regarding tumor progression arose when the results of two randomized, placebo-controlled clinical trials, one involving patients with head and neck cancer undergoing radiotherapy (40) and the other in patients with breast cancer beginning treatment with chemotherapy (41), were reported. In the head and neck trial, an increased rate of locoregional progression was noted in the ESP-treated arm. Although there were significant imbalances in important prognostic factors favoring the placebo group and a substantial number of protocol violations in terms of radiotherapy and follow-up examinations, this study raised legitimate concerns regarding the potential of ESPs to facilitate tumor progression and/or resistance to therapy. In 2005, the breast cancer trial had not been reported except in a very brief letter, but it was clear that there were issues regarding the conduct of the trial (including the eligibility of enrolled patients) and the collection of the baseline prognostic information requisite to balancing baseline prognosis and interpreting the findings of a survival trial in breast cancer, in which prognosis can vary widely. Nevertheless, this trial raised similar concerns.

In parallel laboratory work, investigators reported the detection of EPO-R protein on head and neck (42) and breast (43) cancers, which further raised concerns about the potential for ESPs to enhance resistance to apoptosis and/or induce proliferation of tumor types for which a negative impact on patients in terms of tumor progression or survival had been reported. The majority of laboratory studies that have reported the presence of EPO-R on human tumor cells have used polyclonal antisera raised to a portion of EPO-R; these reagents appear to bind several proteins other than EPO-R, and there is currently no compelling evidence that EPO-R is present on the membranes of human cancer cells and no evidence for functional EPO-R.

These issues were addressed thoroughly by the U.S. Food and Drug Administration and the corporate sponsors of ESPs in a meeting of the Oncology Drug Advisory Committee (ODAC) in May of 2004. The briefing documents and presentation slides are still available on the internet (http://www.fda.gov/ohrms/dockets/ac/04/briefing/4037b2.htm) and represent an excellent resource for the reader interested in exploring these issues in detail. There are two lines of evidence that provide considerable reassurance.

❖ First, as was recognized at the ODAC meeting, both of the trials reporting a negative survival impact were carried out in patients who were not anemic; the goal of therapy was to prevent, as opposed to treat, anemia. It is quite possible that the impacts of increasing hemoglobin levels on tumor biology are different for patients who are anemic at baseline versus patients who have a normal baseline hemoglobin level, with correction of anemia associated with neutral or beneficial effects on tumor outcomes and hemoglobin increases above normal levels having a negative effect.

❖ Second, an independent meta-analysis of randomized trials of ESPs in anemic patients with CIA has been published and shows no negative impact on tumor progression or survival (44). In fact, there is a trend suggesting improved survival in the ESP group (hazard ratio, 0.81; confidence interval, 0.67– 0.99). At present, there is no evidence that ESPs have a negative effect on tumor progression or survival when used to treat, as opposed to prevent, anemia.

The safety of raising hemoglobin levels above normal is not established and should only be undertaken as part of a well-designed and monitored clinical trial. This is the rationale for setting a hemoglobin target of 12 g/dL for cancer patients receiving ESPs and for withholding therapy if the hemoglobin exceeds 13 g/dL.

The second safety issue concerns thrombosis. ESPs are known to increase thrombosis risk in dialysis patients. In randomized trials in cancer patients, a statistically significant increase in thrombotic complications in the ESP-treated group has not been reported. In 2005, pooling of multiple studies increased the power to detect differences in thrombosis rates, and there appears to be an increased incidence of thrombotic complications associated with ESP therapy (45). This is best delineated in the ODAC briefing documents, with the effect observed with all current ESPs and a hazard ratio of 1.3:1.7. What is not clear in the available databases is whether there is a link between hemoglobin response (rapid rate of rise or rise above normal levels) and thrombosis or, alternatively, that thrombosis risk is mediated by a direct effect of ESPs on vascular endothelium and/or platelets (46). Nevertheless, until these issues are resolved, 12 g/dL is a prudent target hemoglobin level, and ESP dose reductions are suggested for patients in whom a rapid rate of hemoglobin rise is observed.

In general, there is a higher risk of thrombosis in cancer patients, with the precise risk depending on the primary cancer site and histology, sites of metastatic disease, anticancer therapy (e.g., tamoxifen, thalidomide), indwelling catheters, and activity level. One of the most consistent predictors of thrombosis is a history of thrombosis. For the population of cancer patients enrolled in randomized trials of ESPs, the observed rate of thrombotic complications has been approximately 3% in the control groups and 5% in the ESP-treated group. The most frequently seen thrombotic complication is catheter-associated thrombosis, but deep venous thrombosis and thromboembolism are also observed. Unless a patient has a history of deep venous thrombosis, full anticoagulation is not necessary when ESP therapy is started. If the patient has a history of deep venous thrombosis, the risk of subsequent thrombosis during cancer treatment is substantial (15%) even if ESP therapy is not started, and a case can be made for anticoagulation regardless of any decision regarding ESP use.

Treatment of Fatigue in the Non-Anemic Cancer Patient

Fatigue is a very common and debilitating symptom in cancer patients. As noted previously, anemia has emerged as an unexpected and highly treatable explanation of fatigue in cancer patients but is responsible for only 15%–20% of the variations in energy level in this patient population. Even in the era of effective erythropoietic agents, fatigue remains a tremendous problem for cancer patients and their caregivers. Frequently, fatigued patients are not anemic, and fatigued anemic patients continue to have some residual fatigue once anemia is successfully treated.

Except for some distinct clinical circumstances in which it is clearly caused by a specific treatment (most notably cranial irradiation and therapy with high-dose interferon or interleukin-2), fatigue in cancer patients is usually gradual in its development and is multifactorial. Unfortunately, the pathophysiology of fatigue is far less well understood than is that of anemia. Fatigue is experienced as debilitating tiredness and loss of energy, usually as part of a larger syndrome that includes varying features:

❖ Depression
❖ Loss of appetite
❖ Cachexia
❖ Debilitation

Evidence is accumulating that cytokines, including tumor necrosis factor, interleukin-1, type 1 interferons, interleukin-6, transforming growth factor β, and interleukin-2, play a central role in this tumor-associated involution syndrome (47). However, because our understanding of the mechanisms underlying tumor involution is rudimentary, the approach to management remains empiric and only marginally successful. The etiology of fatigue in cancer patients is summarized in Figure 5.

Several of the factors contributing to the experience of fatigue by a cancer patient are treatable and are covered in the chapters Chemotherapy-Induced Nausea and Vomiting (CINV), Depression Anxiety, and Cancer Pain Management at the Bedside. It is an important early step in the approach to treatment of the fatigued cancer patient to assess pain control, depression, nausea, sleep disturbances, and nutritional status and implement aggressive interventions. However, as with anemia, some cancer patients debilitated by fatigue do not present with clear features of depression, chemotherapy-induced nausea, or pain and, when these are present, significant fatigue persists after they are treated. These patients with cancer-related fatigue are discussed in the remainder of this chapter.

Description of the Patient with Cancer-Related Fatigue

Although cancer-related fatigue can occur in any oncology setting, it is much more common in patients with certain primary tumor types (lymphoma, Hodgkin's disease, renal cell carcinoma, lung and

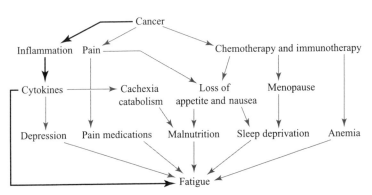

Figure 5
Etiology of fatigue in cancer patients.

pancreatic cancers) or when any cancer is extensive and rapidly progressing or involves the liver. These patients often appear chronically ill, have facial muscle wasting (especially when compared to a past photograph), and complain of severe generalized weakness, night sweats, and low-grade fevers. In less severe cases, only the symptom of overwhelming, debilitating tiredness is present.

Treatment of Cancer-Related Fatigue

The treatment of fatigue that persists after anemia, nausea, pain, and depression have been ruled out or treated is challenging. Although occasional successes are encountered with corticosteroids, nonsteroidal anti-inflammatory drugs (especially in patients with fevers), and antidepressants (especially for fatigue associated with interferon therapy), these interventions are usually not effective. Recently, some success has been reported with central nervous system stimulants. Frequently used drugs are summarized in Table 2.

Although more success is encountered with the agents listed in Table 2 than with any other pharmacologic intervention, there are some caveats:

❖ First, all of these agents may impair the activity of antihypertensive medications and lower seizure threshold; they should be used with caution in patients with serious hypertension or uncontrolled seizures.
❖ Second, there have not been published pivotal clinical trials with any of these agents documenting efficacy for cancer-associated fatigue, and none is approved by the U.S. Food and Drug Administration for this indication.

Modafinil (Provigil®, Cephalon) is used to treat narcolepsy, and methylphenidate (Ritalin®, Novartis) and dexmethylphenidate (Focalin®, Novartis) are used to treat attention deficit disorders. In 2005, a randomized, placebo-controlled trial of dexmethylphenidate for the treatment of cancer related fatigue and cognitive impairment was reported in abstract form (48). The data demonstrated a clear and significant effect on objective validated measures of cancer-related

Table 2. Drugs Used in Treatment of Cancer-Related Fatigue

Brand Name, Manufacturer	Generic Name	Dose	Mechanism	Comments
Provigil®, Cephalon	Modafinil	200 mg PO daily	Nonadrenergic wakefulness promoter	Inhibits CYP2C19 enzyme, increases phenytoin and diazepam levels
Ritalin®, Novartis	Methylphenidate	10 mg PO BID or TID	Activates brainstem and cortex	Inhibits coumarin, phenobarbital, and phenytoin metabolism
Focalin®, Novartis	Dexmethylphenidate	5 mg PO BID titrated to 25 mg PO BID	Activates brainstem and cortex	Inhibits coumarin, phenobarbital, and phenytoin metabolism

fatigue. There was also some improvement in cognitive impairment, which has been reported in cancer patients and frequently coexists with fatigue. These are the best data available for any pharmacologic intervention for this problem to date.

Current pharmacologic interventions may improve but do not eliminate cancer-related fatigue. Hence, an indispensable component of management includes counseling in strategies for living with optimal quality of life and productivity despite tiredness, using strategies such as napping, prioritizing daily activities, and obtaining help with strenuous tasks.

The most obvious opportunity for future improvements in the management of cancer-related fatigue are through a better understanding of the roles of individual cytokines in the development of this syndrome and rationally designed clinical trials of strategies for reversing the pathophysiology, once understood. As an example, early clinical trials of tumor necrosis factor blockade are in progress. Whenever possible, patients with significant cancer-related fatigue should be offered participation in clinical trials.

An algorithm for the management of fatigue in cancer patients is presented in Figure 6.

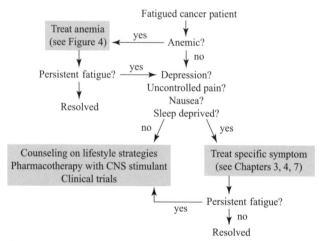

Figure 6
Algorithm for the treatment of fatigue in cancer patients. CNS, central nervous system.

References

1. Stasi R, Abriani L, Beccaglia P, et al. Cancer-related fatigue: evolving concepts in evaluation and treatment. Cancer 2003;98(9):1786–1801.

2. Vogelzang NJ, Breitbart W, Cella D, et al. Patient, caregiver, and oncologist perceptions of cancer-related fatigue: results of a tripart assessment survey. The Fatigue Coalition. Semin Hematol 1997;34(3 Suppl 2):4–12.

3. Curt GA, Breitbart W, Cella D, et al. Impact of cancer-related fatigue on the lives of patients: new findings from the Fatigue Coalition. Oncologist 2000;5(5):353–360.

4. Glaspy J. The impact of epoetin alfa on quality of life during cancer chemotherapy: a fresh look at an old problem. Semin Hematol 1997; 34(3 Suppl 2):20–26.

5. Ludwig H, Fritz E, Kotzmann H, et al. Erythropoietin treatment of anemia associated with multiple myeloma. N Engl J Med 1990;322(24): 1693–1699.

6. Leitgeb C, Pecherstorfer M, Fritz E, et al. Quality of life in chronic anemia of cancer during treatment with recombinant human erythropoietin. Cancer 1994;73(10):2535–2542.

7. Glaspy J, Berg R, Tomita D, et al. Final results of a phase 3, randomized, open-label study of darbepoetin alfa 200 mcg every 2 weeks (Q2W) versus epoetin alfa 40,000 U weekly (QW) in patients with chemotherapy-induced anemia (CIA). Proc Am Soc Clin Oncol 2005;23(16S):760s.

8. Gabrilove JL, Cleeland CS, Livingston RB, et al. Clinical evaluation of once-weekly dosing of epoetin alfa in chemotherapy patients: improvements in hemoglobin and quality of life are similar to three-times-weekly dosing. J Clin Oncol 2001;19(11):2875–2882.

9. Demetri GD, Kris M, Wade J, et al. Quality-of-life benefit in chemotherapy patients treated with epoetin alfa is independent of disease response or tumor type: results from a prospective community oncology study. Procrit Study Group. J Clin Oncol 1998;16(10):3412–3425.

10. Fallowfield L, Gagnon D, Zagari M, et al. Multivariate regression analyses of data from a randomised, double- blind, placebo-controlled study confirm quality of life benefit of epoetin alfa in patients receiving non-platinum chemotherapy. Br J Cancer 2002;87(12):1341–1353.

11. Cella D, Kallich J, McDermott A, et al. The longitudinal relationship of hemoglobin, fatigue and quality of life in anemic cancer patients: results from five randomized clinical trials. Ann Oncol 2004;15(6):979–986.

12. Cella D, Dobrez D, Glaspy J. Control of cancer-related anemia with erythropoietic agents: a review of evidence for improved quality of life and clinical outcomes. Ann Oncol 2003;14(4):511–519.

13. Cella D, Zagari MJ, Vandoros C, et al. Epoetin alfa treatment results in clinically significant improvements in quality of life in anemic cancer patients when referenced to the general population. J Clin Oncol 2003;21(2):366–373.

14. Jones M, Schenkel B, Just J, et al. Epoetin alfa improves quality of life in patients with cancer: results of metaanalysis. Cancer 2004;101(8): 1720–1732.

15. Littlewood TJ, Bajetta E, Nortier JW, et al. Effects of epoetin alfa on hematologic parameters and quality of life in cancer patients receiving nonplatinum chemotherapy: results of a randomized, double-blind, placebo-controlled trial. J Clin Oncol 2001;19(11):2865–2874.

16. Quirt I, Robeson C, Lau CY, et al. Epoetin alfa therapy increases hemoglobin levels and improves quality of life in patients with cancer-related anemia who are not receiving chemotherapy and patients with anemia who are receiving chemotherapy. J Clin Oncol 2001;19(21):4126–4134.

17. Vadhan-Raj S, Mirtsching B, Charu V, et al. Assessment of hematologic effects and fatigue in cancer patients with chemotherapy-induced anemia given darbepoetin alfa every two weeks. J Support Oncol 2003;1(2):131–138.

18. Vansteenkiste J, Pirker R, Massuti B, et al. Double-blind, placebo-controlled, randomized phase III trial of darbepoetin alfa in lung cancer patients receiving chemotherapy. J Natl Cancer Inst 2002;94(16):1211–1220.

19. Miller CB, Jones RJ, Piantadosi S, et al. Decreased erythropoietin response in patients with the anemia of cancer. N Engl J Med 1990; 322(24):1689–1692.

20. Nemeth E, Rivera S, Gabayan V, et al. IL-6 mediates hypoferremia of inflammation by inducing the synthesis of the iron regulatory hormone hepcidin. J Clin Invest 2004;113(9):1271–1276.

21. Rivera S, Liu L, Nemeth E, et al. Hepcidin excess induces the sequestration of iron and exacerbates tumor-associated anemia. Blood 2005;105(4):1797–1802.

22. Weinstein DA, Roy CN, Fleming MD, et al. Inappropriate expression of hepcidin is associated with iron refractory anemia: implications for the anemia of chronic disease. Blood 2002;100(10):3776–3781.

23. Ludwig H, Sundal E, Pecherstorfer M, et al. Recombinant human erythropoietin for the correction of cancer associated anemia with and without concomitant cytotoxic chemotherapy. Cancer 1995;76(11):2319–2329.

24. Smith RE, Tchekmedyian NS, Chan D, et al. A dose- and schedule-finding study of darbepoetin alpha for the treatment of chronic anaemia of cancer. Br J Cancer 2003;88(12):1851–1858.

25. Henry DH, Abels RI. Recombinant human erythropoietin in the treatment of cancer and chemotherapy-induced anemia: results of double-blind and open-label follow-up studies. Semin Oncol 1994;21(2 Suppl 3):21–28.

26. Denton TA, Diamond GA, Matloff JM, et al. Anemia therapy: individual benefit and societal cost. Semin Oncol 1994;21(2 Suppl 3):29–35.

27. Barosi G, Marchetti M, Liberato NL. Cost-effectiveness of recombinant human erythropoietin in the prevention of chemotherapy-induced anaemia. Br J Cancer 1998;78(6):781–787.

28. Marchetti M, Barosi G. Clinical and economic impact of epoetins in cancer care. Pharmacoeconomics 2004;22(16):1029–1045.

29. Ortega A, Dranitsaris G, Puodziunas AL. What are cancer patients willing to pay for prophylactic epoetin alfa? A cost-benefit analysis. Cancer 1998;83(12):2588–2596.

30. Rizzo JD, Lichtin AE, Woolf SH, et al. Use of epoetin in patients with cancer: evidence-based clinical practice guidelines of the American Society of Clinical Oncology and the American Society of Hematology. Blood 2002;100(7):2303–2320.

31. Lyman G, Glaspy JA. At what hemoglobin level should erythropoietic therapy be initiated for chemotherapy-induced anemia? A systematic review. Cancer 2005 (in press).

32. Crawford J, Cella D, Cleeland CS, et al. Relationship between changes in hemoglobin level and quality of life during chemotherapy in anemic cancer patients receiving epoetin alfa therapy. Cancer 2002;95(4):888–895.

33. Glaspy JA. The development of erythropoietic agents in oncology. Expert Opin Emerg Drugs 2005;10(3):1–15.

34. Bokemeyer C, Aapro MS, Courdi A, et al. EORTC guidelines for the use of erythropoietic proteins in anaemic patients with cancer. Eur J Cancer 2004;40(15):2201–2216.

35. Anonymous. Cancer and treatment-related anemia. NCCN Practice Guidelines in Oncology 2004;2:ANEM 1–ANEM 5.

36. Roy CN, Andrews NC. Anemia of inflammation: the hepcidin link. Curr Opin Hematol 2005;12(2):107–111.

37. Auerbach M, Ballard H, Trout JR, et al. Intravenous iron optimizes the response to recombinant human erythropoietin in cancer patients with chemotherapy-related anemia: a multicenter, open-label, randomized trial. J Clin Oncol 2004;22(7):1301–1307.

38. Henry D, Dahl N, Auerbach D, et al. Intravenous ferric gluconate (FG) for increasing response to epoetin (EPO) in patients with anemia of cancer chemotherapy—results of a multi-center, randomized trial. Blood 2004;104(11):abstract 3696.

39. Brugnara C. Iron deficiency and erythropoiesis: new diagnostic approaches. Clin Chem 2003;49(10):1573–1578.

40. Henke M, Laszig R, Rube C, et al. Erythropoietin to treat head and neck cancer patients with anaemia undergoing radiotherapy: randomised, double-blind, placebo-controlled trial. Lancet 2003;362(9392):1255–1260.

41. Leyland-Jones B. Breast cancer trial with erythropoietin terminated unexpectedly. Lancet Oncol 2003;4(8):459–460.

42. Arcasoy MO, Amin K, Chou SC, et al. Erythropoietin and erythropoietin receptor expression in head and neck cancer: relationship to tumor hypoxia. Clin Cancer Res 2005;11(1):20–27.

43. Acs G, Acs P, Beckwith SM, et al. Erythropoietin and erythropoietin receptor expression in human cancer. Cancer Res 2001;61(9):3561–3565.

44. Bohlius J, Langensiepen S, Schwarzer G, et al. Recombinant human erythropoietin and overall survival in cancer patients: results of a comprehensive meta-analysis. J Natl Cancer Inst 2005;97(7):490–498.

45. Bohlius J, Langensiepen S, Schwarzer G, et al. Erythropoietin for patients with malignant disease (review). The Cochrane Library 2005;1:1–163.

46. Stohlawetz PJ, Dzirlo L, Hergovich N, et al. Effects of erythropoietin on platelet reactivity and thrombopoiesis in humans. Blood 2000; 95(9):2983–2989.

47. Illman J, Corringham R, Robinson D, et al. Are inflammatory cytokines the common link between cancer-associated cachexia and depression? J Support Oncol 2005;3(1):37–50.

48. Lower E, Fleishman S, Cooper A, et al. A phase III, randomized placebo-controlled trial of the safety and efficacy of d-MPH as new treatment of fatigue and "chemobrain" in adult cancer patients. Proc Am Soc Clin Oncol 2005;23(16s):729s (abst 8000).

Febrile Neutropenia

Gary H. Lyman, MD, MPH, FRCP (Edin), and
Nicole M. Kuderer, MD

Background

Myelosuppression and Febrile Neutropenia

Myelosuppression remains the leading cause of dose-limiting toxicity associated with systemic cancer chemotherapy. Fever in the setting of neutropenia or febrile neutropenia (FN) is defined as a single temperature of ≥38.3°C (101°F) or a sustained temperature of ≥38.0°C (100.4°F) for at least 1 hour in a patient with an absolute neutrophil count (ANC) <500 cells/mm^3 or <1,000 cells/mm^3 and likely to fall below 500 cells/mm^3 (Table 1) (1). Early studies demonstrated that, even in the absence of clinical signs or symptoms, most patients with FN have occult bacterial infections with a high risk of early mortality unless treated with immediate antibiotics. Therefore, FN is considered a true medical emergency, generally prompting immediate hospitalization for evaluation and the administration of empiric broad-spectrum antibiotics (2). It must be noted that elderly neutropenic patients and those receiving immunosuppressive medications may not develop fever and may, in fact, become hypothermic. Nonetheless, such patients should be placed on empiric antibiotics if symptoms or signs of infection are present or clinical deterioration occurs.

Table 1. Definitions

Fever is defined as
A single oral temperature of ≥38.3°C (101°F)
or
A temperature of ≥38.0°C (100.4°F) for a least 1 h
Neutropenia is defined as
An absolute neutrophil count of <500 cells/mm^3 (grade 4)
or
An absolute neutrophil count of <1,000 cells/mm^3 (grade 3 or 4), with a predicted decrease to <500 cells/mm^3

Risk of Febrile Neutropenia

The risk of FN has been shown to increase in proportion to the severity and duration of neutropenia (Figure 1). Bodey and colleagues (3) also demonstrated that patients with documented infection, most notably related to gram-negative bacteremia, often experienced a rapid and fatal outcome without antibiotic therapy while awaiting culture results. These observations led to the current policy of emergent hospitalization of patients with FN for immediate evaluation and administration of empiric, broad-spectrum antibiotics, considerably reducing the mortality associated with FN.

Risk Factors for Febrile Neutropenia

The risk of FN varies with the type and intensity of the treatment regimen and delivered dose intensity as well as host-related factors, such as age, the type of cancer, and various comorbid conditions. It has been shown that the risk of hematologic complications, including FN, is significantly under-reported in randomized controlled trials (RCTs) (4). A number of efforts to identify risk factors for the occurrence of FN or its consequences in those with established FN have been reported. A recent systematic review of published studies of risk models for FN and its consequences has been reported (5). Shown in Figure 2 are those characteristics reported in two or more studies to be significant independent risk factors for FN in multivariate analysis. Risk factors for FN are summarized as follows (6):

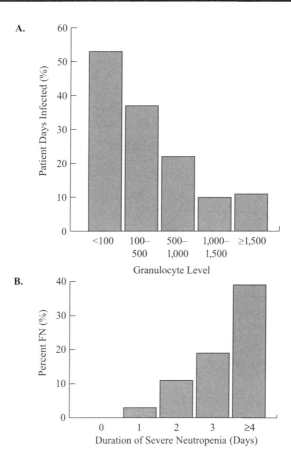

Figure 1
A: Graphic representation of the relationship between the severity of neutropenia and the proportion of days spent with infection. **B:** A similar relationship is observed between the duration of severe neutropenia and the risk of febrile neutropenia (FN). (From Bodey GP, Buckley M, Sathe YS, et al. Quantitative relationships between circulating leukocytes and infection in patients with acute leukemia. Ann Int Med 1966;64:328–340, with permission.)

Treatment related

- ❖ Previous history of severe neutropenia with similar chemotherapy
- ❖ Type of chemotherapy (anthracyclines)
- ❖ Planned relative dose intensity >80%

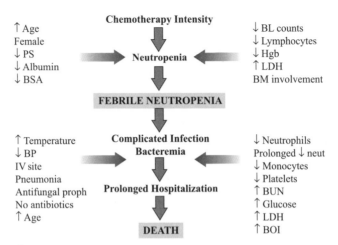

Figure 2
Risk factors for chemotherapy-induced febrile neutropenia **(top)** and the risk of serious medical consequences, including long length of stay and mortality **(bottom)** identified in two or more published multivariate risk models. BL, baseline; BM, bone marrow; BOI, burden of illness; BP, blood pressure; BSA, body surface area; BUN, blood urea nitrogen; Hgb, hemoglobin; LDH, lactate dehydrogenase; neut, neutrophil; proph, prophylactic; PS, performance status. (From Lyman GH, Lyman CH, Agboola O. Risk models for predicting chemotherapy-induced neutropenia. Oncologist 2005;10:427–437, with permission.)

❖ Pre-existing neutropenia or lymphocytopenia
❖ Extensive prior chemotherapy
❖ Concurrent or prior radiation therapy to marrow containing bone

Patient related

❖ Increasing age
❖ Female gender
❖ Poor performance status
❖ Poor nutritional status (e.g., low albumin)
❖ Decreased immune function

Cancer related

❖ Bone marrow involvement with tumor
❖ Advanced cancer
❖ Elevated lactate dehydrogenase (lymphoma)

Conditions associated with risk of serious infection

- ❖ Open wounds
- ❖ Active tissue infection

Comorbidities

- ❖ Chronic obstructive pulmonary disease
- ❖ Cardiovascular disease
- ❖ Liver disease (elevated bilirubin, alkaline phosphatase)
- ❖ Diabetes mellitus
- ❖ Low baseline hemoglobin

Timing of Febrile Neutropenia

The risk of the initial episode of FN appears to be greatest during the first cycle of chemotherapy when the majority of patients receive full-dose intensity often without FN prophylaxis (Figure 3) (7,8). Early neutropenic complications generally prompt chemotherapy dose reductions, treatment delays, or the addition of a myeloid growth factor in subsequent cycles. However, in the absence of major dose reductions, treatment delays, or the addition of prophylactic myeloid growth factors or antibiotics, the risk of FN is the same or greater with subsequent cycles of the same regimen. Therefore, the majority of patients who experience an initial episode of FN experience additional episodes on subsequent cycles under such circumstances.

Complications of Febrile Neutropenia

Episodes of FN are associated with substantial morbidity, mortality, and cost, as well as dose reductions and treatment delays that may compromise the delivery of full-dose intensity.

Morbidity

- ❖ FN compromises patient quality of life through the requirement for hospitalization, the performance of multiple tests, and the frequent delivery of intravenous antibiotics as well as

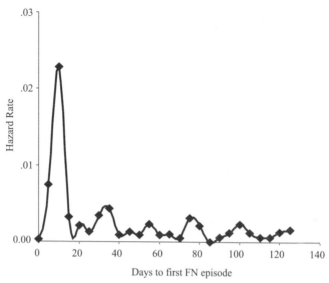

Figure 3
Hazard plot of febrile neutropenia (FN) in 577 patients with non-Hodgkin's lymphoma treated with cyclophosphamide, hydroxydaunomycin, vincristine (Oncovin), and prednisone chemotherapy. (From Lyman GH, Morrison VA, Dale DC, et al. Risk of febrile neutropenia among patients with intermediate-grade non-Hodgkin's lymphoma receiving CHOP chemotherapy. Leuk Lymphoma 2003;44:2069–2076, with permission.)

the general sense of ill health associated with fever or other signs of infection. In addition, the FN patient is at increased risk for experiencing infectious complications and worsening of comorbid conditions.

Mortality

❖ Risk of mortality: The risk of mortality associated with FN has been variably reported from 0% to 20% with even higher mortality rates among patients with comorbid conditions and infectious complications, including septic shock (9–16).

❖ Randomized controlled trials: The mortality rates reported in RCTs of antibiotics or myeloid growth factors may underestimate the risk of infection-related mortality owing to the highly selected nature of patients in such trials compared to the greater frequency of infection-related mortality reported in the general cancer population.

❖ Septicemia: Documented sepsis reflects a systemic inflammatory response to bacteremia, potentially leading to septic shock with hypotension, oliguria, lactic acidosis, and ultimately multiorgan dysfunction (9). The incidence of sepsis in patients with FN has not been well characterized but is estimated to be in the range of around 20%–40% (10,11). In a consecutive series of 438 patients with neutropenia and bacteremia, the overall mortality was 24% with significantly increased risk associated with shock at presentation, pneumonia, uncontrolled cancer, and no prophylactic antibiotics (12).

❖ Septic shock: Malik et al. (13) reported that the mortality rate associated with FN in patients presenting in shock is 82%. Similarly, a 30-day mortality of 54% has been observed in critically ill patients with FN (14).

❖ Polymicrobial bacteremia: Polymicrobial bacteremia in neutropenic patients continues to be associated with high mortality rates. Although a mortality rate of 5% has been observed in those with *Pseudomonas* bacteremia as the only organism, 50% of patients died when *Pseudomonas* was a component of a polymicrobial bacteremia (15).

❖ Pneumonia: Carratala et al. (16) reported that despite prompt treatment with appropriate antibiotics, neutropenic cancer patients with pneumonia experienced a 54% mortality rate when associated with gram-negative bacteremia and 53% when accompanied by gram-positive bacteremia.

Costs

❖ The costs associated with FN are primarily determined by the complexity and duration of hospitalization.

❖ Average lengths of hospital stay with FN from randomized controlled trials and multiple institution surveys range from 7 to 11 days, with longer stays in patients with leukemia than in those with solid tumors or lymphoma (17).

❖ Average total costs range from $10,000 to $20,000 per episode depending on the type of malignancy, intensity of treatment, and presence of comorbidities and infectious complications (17).

Reduced Chemotherapy Dose Intensity

❖ Perhaps the most concerning complication of FN is the impact on delivered dose intensity in patients receiving chemotherapy with responsive malignancies, potentially compromising long-term disease control and curability. Substantially reduced chemotherapy dose intensity associated with FN has been observed in more than one-half of patients receiving chemotherapy for early-stage breast cancer or aggressive non-Hodgkin's lymphoma (18,19).

Evaluation of the Patient with Febrile Neutropenia

Initial Evaluation

Patients with FN should be immediately admitted, evaluated, and started on broad-spectrum antibacterial therapy within 1 hour of presentation. Table 2 provides a checklist of the recommended sequence of initial and subsequent management steps in the patient with FN. The initial evaluation should include a careful history, detailed physical examination, and appropriate radiologic and laboratory examinations, as well as blood, wound, and other cultures with gram stains when indicated. Rectal and vaginal examinations and manipulations should generally be avoided unless absolutely necessary. Infection in the patient with neutropenia may not manifest common signs and symptoms of infection related to leukocyte infiltration, for example, redness, swelling, pain, warmth, pus, nuchal rigidity, cerebrospinal fluid pleocytosis, pyuria and pulmonary infiltrates on chest radiograph.

Cultures

Cultures should be sampled from every possible site of infection, including two sets of blood cultures, intravenous lines or other catheters, sputum, urine with urinalysis, and skin lesions. In patients with diarrhea, stool cultures are indicated, including *Clostridium difficile* antigen assay. An initial series of blood cultures should be followed by repeat cultures at reasonable intervals in persistently febrile neutropenic patients. It must be kept in mind that cultures will remain negative in more than half of patients with FN despite the likely infectious etiology of the fever.

Table 2.   Febrile Neutropenia Management Check List

Initial evaluation (<1 h)

History

1. Careful history with focus on new symptoms and sites that are commonly infected, especially symptoms of upper and lower respiratory tract, upper and lower GI tract, GU tract, skin and soft tissue changes, mental status or other neurologic changes and pain, symptoms of hypotension, dehydration, and bleeding.

2. Timing and type of chemotherapy, recent antibiotics, or growth factor usage.

3. Recent infections, procedures, catheter placements, or surgeries.

4. History of MRSA, VRE, HIV, viral hepatitis, or fungal infections; sick contacts or other infectious exposures (TB, pets) and travel history.

5. Allergies and recent changes in medications; comorbid conditions.

Physical examination

1. A complete and detailed physical examination should be performed, including vital signs; oropharynx; periodontium; sinuses; ears; ocular fundi; mental status changes and meningismus; lungs; abdomen; change in or new cardiac murmur; skin changes especially around fingernails, perianal, and GU areas; recent surgical and other procedure sites including indwelling catheter sites.

2. Rectal and vaginal examinations and manipulations should generally be avoided unless absolutely necessary. It is generally understood that infections in the patient with neutropenia may not manifest common signs and symptoms associated with infections, i.e., leukocyte infiltration (e.g., redness, swelling, pain, warmth, pus, nuchal rigidity, cerebrospinal fluid pleocytosis, pyuria, pulmonary infiltrates).

Laboratory evaluation

1. Complete blood count and differential.

2. Two sets of blood cultures from separate sites and isolator system cultures as indicated.

3. Cultures and gram stains from other concerning sites of infection, including urine, sputum, stool, skin, and catheters.

4. Evaluate for need of lumbar puncture and viral culture.

Radiologic imaging

1. Chest radiograph in most patients.

(continued)

Table 2. *Continued*

Therapy/management

    1. Appropriate empiric broad-spectrum antibiotics (see Table 4); important to give after blood cultures obtained but within 1 h of assessment.

    2. Intravenous fluid.

    3. Initiate neutropenic precautions (see local institutional guidelines).

Additional evaluation (1–6 h)

History and physical examination

    1. Finalize if not yet finished.

Laboratory evaluation

    1. Complete metabolic profile, including renal and liver function.

    2. Coagulation studies if bleeding, low platelets, or concern for bleeding diathesis.

    3. Urine analysis and rest of necessary cultures if not already done.

    4. If diarrhea is present, get stool cultures ± *Clostridium difficile* toxin immunoassay.

Radiologic imaging

    1. Additional imaging, such as ultrasound or computerized tomography, when symptoms or signs of local infection justify it.

    2. Computerized tomography often reveals pulmonary nodules or infiltration in patients with persistent fever despite a normal chest x-ray (42).

Therapy/management

    1. Additional antibiotics if indicated.

    2. Consider colony-stimulating growth factors in patients at increased risk (Table 7).

    3. Supportive care as indicated, low threshold for more intensive care.

    4. Monitor vital signs closely.

Follow-up (<24 h)

History

    1. Monitor chief complaints and detailed review of systems.

    2. Red flags: altered mental status and new neurologic symptoms, respiratory compromise and increased oxygen need, acute pain, bleeding, hypotension.

Physical examination

    1. Detailed physical examination.

Table 2. *Continued*

Laboratory evaluation

1. Follow-up blood counts, renal function, and other abnormal laboratory results.
2. Follow-up culture data.

Imaging

1. Reassess need for further imaging.

Therapy/management

1. Supportive care as indicated, low threshold for more intensive care.
2. Monitor vital signs closely.

Further evaluation (>24 h)

History

1. Monitor closely any changes in symptoms.

Physical examination

1. Daily detailed physical examination, especially vital signs, oropharynx, lungs, abdomen, skin, and catheters.

Laboratory evaluation

1. Daily complete blood counts and differential (to monitor neutropenia).
2. Follow renal function, hepatic function, and other abnormal laboratory values at least every 3 days (to monitor potential end organ damage).
3. Follow-up culture data, repeat blood cultures if continued fever, other cultures as clinically indicated.
4. Consider need for additional studies, e.g., bronchoscopy.

Imaging

1. Reassess need for further imaging, especially if fever persists for several days despite appropriate therapy.

Therapy/management

1. Reassess appropriateness and length of antibiotic therapy.
2. Reassess need for colony-stimulating factors.
3. Supportive care as indicated, low threshold for more intensive care if remains neutropenic.
4. Monitor vitals signs closely.

GI, gastrointestinal; GU, genitourinary; HIV, human immunodeficiency virus; MRSA, methicillin-resistant *Staphylococcus aureus*; TB, tuberculosis; VRE, vancomycin-resistant enterococcus.

Common Sites of Infection

- ❖ Central nervous system
- ❖ Head and neck: mucositis, gingivitis, sinusitis
- ❖ Chest: pneumonia (bacterial, fungal, viral, parasitic)
- ❖ Gastrointestinal: esophagitis, typhlitis, *C. difficile*, perirectal abscess, perianal cellulitis
- ❖ Genitourinary: urinary tract infection
- ❖ Skin: cellulitis, vascular access device, tunnel infection (erythema or tenderness >2 cm from catheter exit site)

Infectious Agents

Common Infectious Agents

Documented infections are most commonly bacterial, although fungal, mycobacterial, viral, and parasitic etiologies should be considered. In addition to myelosuppression and neutropenia, cancer patients exhibit several other factors that further increase their predisposition to infections (20):

- ❖ Intravenous catheters and other devices
- ❖ Mucositis/tissue damage
- ❖ Lymphopenia
- ❖ Cellular and humoral immunodeficiency
- ❖ Chemotherapeutic regimen
- ❖ Adrenal corticosteroid therapy
- ❖ Bone marrow transplantation
- ❖ Tumor involvement of bone marrow
- ❖ Acute leukemia
- ❖ Antimicrobial prophylaxis
- ❖ Colonization
- ❖ Environmental sources
- ❖ Seasonal exposures

The majority of infections in patients with FN arise from a patient's own endogenous flora. Table 3 lists common and uncommon infectious organisms found in febrile neutropenic patients.

Table 3. Organisms Causing Infection in Neutropenic Patients

Common	Uncommon
Gram positive	Gram positive
Staphylococcus epidermidis	*Enterococcus*
Staphylococcus aureus	*Corynebacterium jeikeium*
Streptococcus viridans	*Stomatococcus mucilaginosus*
Streptococcus pneumoniae	*Clostridium* spp.
Gram negative	Gram negative
Escherichia coli	*Stenotrophomonas maltophilia*
Klebsiella spp.	*Capnocytophaga* sp.
Pseudomonas aeruginosa	*Acinetobacter* sp.
Enterobacter spp.	
Serratia marcescens	
Fungi	Fungi
Candida spp.	*Mucorales*
Aspergillus spp.	*Fusarium* spp.
	Trichosporon beigelii
	Blastoschizomyces capitatus
Viruses	Viruses
Herpes simplex	Cytomegalovirus
Respiratory syncytial virus	Influenza

Modified from Abeloff MD, Armitage JO, Niederhuber JE, et al., eds. Clinical oncology, 3rd ed. Philadelphia: Elsevier Churchill Livingstone, 2004.

Bacterial Organisms

❖ The most common offending bacterial organisms are gram-positive cocci, including coagulase positive and negative *Staphylococcus*, and *Streptococcus pneumoniae*, as well as other streptococci.

❖ The most common gram-negative bacteria are *Escherichia coli*, *Klebsiella*, *Pseudomonas*, and *Enterobacter*.

❖ Less common bacterial organisms include *Proteus*, *Haemophilus*, *Listeria*, *Serratia*, and various anaerobic bacteria.

Fungal Organisms

❖ Common fungal organisms in patients with FN include *Aspergillus*, *Candida albicans*, and other *Candida* species.

Less common fungi include *Cryptococcus, Histoplasma*, and *Coccidioides*.

❖ Fungal infections are more likely to occur later in the treatment course after repeated episodes of FN and extensive exposure to antibiotics.

Viral Organisms

❖ Common viral etiologies include the Herpes complex, *Cytomegalovirus*, and *Enterovirus*.

Parasitic Infections

❖ The most common parasitic infection is due to *Pneumocystis carinii*.

Antibiotic-Resistant Organisms

❖ The increasing emergence of antibiotic-resistant organisms, including methicillin- or oxacillin-resistant *Staphylococcus aureus*, vancomycin-resistant enterococcus and vancomycin-resistant coagulase-negative staphylococci, has been of considerable concern. Such changing patterns of antibiotic sensitivity, as well as the greater frequency of gram-positive organisms in patients with FN, appears to relate to the frequent use of prophylactic antibiotics, as well as the frequent use of venous access devices.

Empiric Antibiotic Therapy

Empiric broad-spectrum antibiotics should be started within 1 hour of presentation with FN, after acquisition of cultures, without waiting for the results of testing.

Empiric Antibiotic Regimens

Empiric therapy options for FN include broad-spectrum antibiotics with or without a myeloid growth factor. Multiple empiric antibiotic regimens have been demonstrated to be effective, with no single regimen demonstrated to be clearly superior to others. The choice of empiric antibiotics depends on institutional experience, sensitivity patterns, and the clinical status of the patient. Owing to the demonstrated high risk for early mortality associated with untreated gram-negative septicemia, empiric regimens always provide coverage for gram-negative bacilli, especially *Pseudomonas aeruginosa*.

Guidelines for Empiric Antibiotics in Febrile Neutropenia

Table 4 summarizes the 2002 guidelines of the Infectious Disease Society of America (IDSA) for the use of antimicrobial agents in cancer patients with FN (2). Initial therapy in the uncomplicated patient may involve monotherapy, for example, cefepime, ceftazidime, imipenem-cilastatin, and meropenem. Ceftazidime has been associated with suboptimal treatment of resistant streptococci compared to other monotherapy options. In more complicated cases, combination therapy is generally preferred, including an aminoglycoside combined with either a semisynthetic antipseudomonal penicillin (piperacillin-tazobactam or ticarcillin-clavulanate), an antipseudomonal cephalosporin (cefepime or ceftazidime), or a carbapenem (imipenem-cilastatin or meropenem). The need to modify therapy and evidence of increasing antibiotic resistance may limit confidence in monotherapy at certain institutions. When a specific organism has been identified or is suspected, the antibiotic regimen should include optimal coverage for that organism while maintaining broad coverage for other unidentified but potentially serious organisms.

Vancomycin Usage

Vancomycin should be avoided in the initial empirical therapy except for patients at high risk of serious gram-positive infections because of the emergence of vancomycin-resistant organisms. Table 5 describes the guidelines for appropriate vancomycin usage as recommended by the Centers for Disease Control and Prevention and the IDSA.

Table 4. 2002 Infectious Disease Society of America Guidelines for the Use of Antimicrobial Agents in Neutropenic Patients with Cancer: Executive Summary

Initial antibiotic therapy
  Oral therapy for low-risk adults only
    Ciprofloxacin plus amoxicillin-clavulanate
  Monotherapy without vancomycin
    Cefepime, ceftazidime, imipenem, or meropenem
  Dual therapy without vancomycin
    Aminoglycoside plus antipseudomonal β-lactam, cephalosporin (cefepime or ceftazidime), or carbapenem
  Vancomycin should be added to either monotherapy or dual therapy only if criteria in Table 5 are met

Afebrile within 3–5 days of treatment
  If etiology identified, adjust to most appropriate treatment
  If no etiology identified
    Low risk: change to oral antibiotics [ciprofloxacin/amoxicillin-clavulanate (adults), cefixime (children)] after 48 h
    High risk: continue same intravenous drugs

Persistent fever during first 3–5 days of treatment
  Reassess on day 3
    If no change, continue antibiotics; stop vancomycin if cultures are negative
    If progressive disease, change antibiotics
    If febrile after day 5, consider adding an antifungal drug with or without changes in antibiotics

Duration of antibiotic therapy
  Afebrile by day 3
    If ANC ≥500/mm^3 for 2 days, stop antibiotics if there is no site of infection or positive cultures
    If ANC <500/mm^3 by day 7
      Low risk: stop when afebrile for 5–7 days
      High risk: continue antibiotics

Persistent fever on day 3
  If ANC ≥500/mm^3, stop 4–5 days after ANC is ≥500/mm^3 and reassess
  If ANC <500/mm^3, continue for 2 more wk, reassess and stop if no site identified

ANC, absolute neutrophil count.
Adapted from Hughes WT, Armstrong D, Bodey GP, et al. 2002 Guidelines for the use of antimicrobial agents in neutropenic patients with cancer. Clin Infect Dis 2002; 34:730–751.

Table 5. Appropriate Use of Vancomycin

Inclusion of vancomycin in the initial empirical antibiotic regimen may be indicated for specific patients with the following clinical findings:

Clinically suspected, serious catheter-related infection

Blood culture is positive for gram-positive bacteria before final identification and susceptibility testing

Substantial mucosal damage and high risk for infection with penicillin-resistant *Streptococcus viridans* (especially patients with preceding prophylaxis with quinolone antibiotics or trimethoprim-sulfamethoxazole)

Known colonization with penicillin/cephalosporin-resistant pneumococci or methicillin-resistant *Staphylococcus aureus*

Hypotension or other cardiovascular impairment without identified pathogen

Reassess the appropriateness of vancomycin therapy in 2–3 days after specific culture data and sensitivities are available.

From Centers for Disease Control. Recommendations for preventing the spread of vancomycin resistance. Recommendations of the Hospital Infections Control Practices Advisory Committee (HICPAC). MMWR Morb Mortal Wkly Rep 1995;44(RR12):1–13.

Antifungal Therapy

Owing to the high prevalence of disseminated fungal infection in autopsy series, empiric antifungal therapy should be considered in the persistently febrile patient despite adequate empiric antibacterial therapy for 5–7 days. Newer and less-toxic antifungals, such as voriconazole, caspofungin, and itraconazole, have largely replaced amphotericin as the empiric antifungal agents of choice. Fluconazole should generally not be used for empiric antifungal coverage owing to emerging resistance and its ineffectiveness against several organisms, including *Aspergillus* and various *Candida* species.

Duration of Antibiotic Therapy

The recommended duration of antibiotic treatment depends on the results of the initial evaluation and cultures, as well as on the clinical response to therapy, including fever resolution and neutrophil recovery (Table 6).

Table 6. Specific Suggested Duration of Therapy

Skin/soft tissue: 7–14 days

Bloodstream infection (uncomplicated)
  Gram-negative: 10–14 days
  Gram-positive: 7–14 days
  Staphylococcus aureus: 2 wk
  Yeast: > 2 wk

Sinusitis: 14–21 days

Pneumonia: 14–21 days

Fungal (mold and yeast)
  Continue therapy until there is clinical, microbiologic, and radiologic resolution of infection and resolution of neutropenia

Viral
  Herpes simplex virus: 7–10 days
    Acyclovir, valacyclovir, or famciclovir
  Varicella-zoster virus: 7–10 days
    Acyclovir, valacyclovir, or famciclovir
  Cytomegalovirus: 21 days
    Ganciclovir (pneumonia: add IV immunoglobulin)
    Foscarnet
    Consider suppressive antiviral therapy for 2–4 wk after the completion of cytomegalovirus infection treatment
  For seasonal respiratory viruses use pathogen-specific regimens

Modified from National Comprehensive Cancer Network. Practice guidelines in oncology. Fever and neutropenia. v.1.2005. Available at: http//www.nccn.org/professionals/physician_gls/PDF/fever.pdf. Accessed April 15, 2005.

Afebrile within 3–5 Days

❖ Patients who defervesce rapidly without a specific organism identified should be continued on antibiotics through the period of neutrophil recovery or for at least 5–7 days in low-risk individuals (Figure 4).

❖ When a specific organism has been identified, appropriate directed therapy is essential for a standard period of time, for example, 7–14 days dependent on the site of infection and

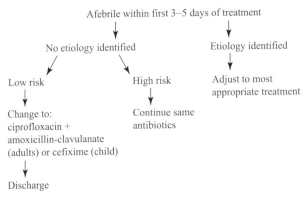

Figure 4
Guide for management of patients who become afebrile in the first 3–5 days of initial antibiotic therapy. (From Infectious Diseases Society of America. 2002 Guidelines for the use of antimicrobial agents in neutropenic patients with cancer. Clin Infect Dis 2002;34:730–751, with permission.)

infectious organism (see Table 6), while still maintaining broad coverage during the neutropenic period.

❖ Cultures remain negative in the majority of patients. In such circumstances, treatment may generally be stopped after 7 days in patients who become afebrile and recover ANC counts >1,000/mm^3.

Persistent Fever for 3–5 Days

❖ In neutropenic patients with persistent fever after 3–5 days, the antibiotic coverage should be reevaluated, including the addition of vancomycin when appropriate.

❖ Persistent fever beyond any alteration of antibacterial therapy should prompt consideration of antifungal coverage (Figure 5).

Persistent Neutropenia

❖ Persistently neutropenic patients should be continued on antibiotics for 7–14 days dependent on the early disappearance of fever.

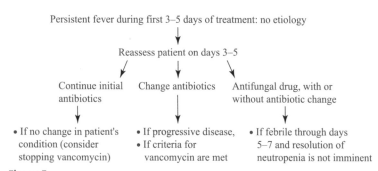

Figure 5
Guide for management of patients with persistent fever after 3–5 days of treatment with negative cultures. (From Infectious Diseases Society of America. 2002 Guidelines for the use of antimicrobial agents in neutropenic patients with cancer. Clin Infect Dis 2002;34:730–751, with permission.)

❖ Persistently febrile patients should be evaluated for fungal infections and other causes of fever with consideration of a trial off antibiotics after 14 days if no infectious site has been identified. They should be closely monitored for recurrence of symptoms or signs of infection.

Catheter Infection

❖ Evidence of tunnel infection or persistent positive cultures from central lines should prompt catheter removal. Many other catheter site infections may be treated with intravenous antibiotics without line removal.

Outpatient Management of Febrile Neutropenia

Although low-risk patients are considered for early discharge and may be treated as outpatients at a number of institutions, the precise role of ambulatory treatment remains to be defined. The limited accuracy of available risk models and the infrastructure costs needed for implementation, as well as issues related to competence, proximity, caretaker availability, and patient anxiety, remain. Outpatient management of FN should be limited to low-risk patients, who are monitored closely for clinical deterioration requiring urgent readmission.

Risk Assessment in Patients with Febrile Neutropenia

High-Risk Febrile Neutropenic Patients

❖ A variety of risk factors for serious medical complications, including death in patients with established FN, have been reported (Table 7; see Figure 2).

❖ Risk factors include the development of FN as an inpatient; hypotension; sepsis; various comorbidities, including cardiovascular and pulmonary disease, leukemia or lymphoma diagnosis; age >65; the severity and duration of neutropenia; prior fungal infection; visceral organ involvement; organ dysfunction; and uncontrolled malignancy (21).

Low-Risk Febrile Neutropenic Patients

❖ In an effort to identify low-risk individuals for possible outpatient management, the Multinational Association of Supportive Care of Cancer (MASCC) identified independent factors at the time of presentation with FN among 756 cancer patients (22). A risk score was designed based on multivariate analysis (Table 8).

❖ In the validation population, a risk score ≥21 identified low-risk patients for serious medical complications, including death. Although the MASCC Index is used to identify low-risk patients, the model has limited test performance, with an overall misclassification rate of 30% [95% confidence interval (CI), 25–34] and 32% (95% CI, 22–43) of patients experiencing serious medical complications labeled by the model as low risk (22).

Therapeutic Use of Myeloid Growth Factors

❖ Guidelines have generally not recommended the routine use of the CSFs in the treatment of established FN (2,23). However, treatment with CSFs has been shown to reduce the duration of severe neutropenia, and they are sometimes considered in critically ill patients, especially those with sepsis, pneumonia, or organ dysfunction.

Table 7.   Risk Factors for Adverse Consequences/Death from Febrile Neutropenia

Hematologic complications

    Severe and prolonged neutropenia

    Anemia

    Thrombocytopenia, monocytopenia

Increasing age

Cancer related

    Leukemia

    Lymphoma

    Lung cancer

    Other advanced or uncontrolled cancer

Comorbidities

    Cardiovascular disease

    Chronic obstructive pulmonary disease

    Renal failure

    Liver disease

    Cerebrovascular

    Pulmonary embolism

    Diabetes mellitus

Infectious complications

    High temperature

    Hypotension (shock, hypovolemia, tachycardia)

    Sepsis (gram negative, gram positive, polymicrobial)

    Pneumonia

    Fungal infection

    IV site infection

    Antifungal prophylaxis

Adapted from Crawford J, Althaus B, Armitage J, et al. Myeloid growth factors. J Natl Compr Canc Netw 2005;3:549–555.

❖ A recent Cochrane meta-analysis of 12 RCTs of therapeutic CSFs as an adjunct to empiric antibiotics in patients with established FN has been reported (24). In addition to the expected reduction in the time to neutrophil recovery across trials ($P <.00001$), the investigators observed significant reduc-

Table 8. Multinational Association of Supportive Care of Cancer Scoring Index Identifying Low-Risk Febrile Neutropenic Patients[a]

Characteristics	Score
Extent of illness	
No/mild symptoms	5
Moderate symptoms	3
No hypotension	5
No COPD	4
Solid tumor or no fungal infection	4
No dehydration	3
Outpatient at onset of fever	3
Age <60 yr	2

COPD, chronic obstructive pulmonary disease.
[a]Score range 0–26: A risk score ≥21 indicates a low-risk patient for medical complications and mortality (26).
Adapted from Klastersky J, Paesmans M, Rubenstein EB, et al. The Multinational Association for Supportive Care in Cancer risk index: a multinational scoring system for identifying low-risk febrile neutropenic cancer patients. J Clin Oncol 2000;18:3038–3051.

tions in the length of hospitalization ($P = .0006$) and infection-related mortality ($P = .05$).

❖ The use of the CSFs should be considered in higher-risk patients hospitalized with FN at increased risk, including the elderly, those with significant comorbidities (lung, heart, renal, liver disease), those with infectious complications (hypotension, documented sepsis, pneumonia), and those with very severe (ANC <100/mm^3) or prolonged neutropenia (>7 days).

Prophylaxis of Febrile Neutropenia

Early Efforts

Efforts to reduce the risk of FN associated with myelosuppression have ranged from prophylactic antibiotics and hematopoietic growth factors to total protective isolation with sterilization of air, food, water, and patient. Protective isolation with laminar airflow filtration is frequently used in patients undergoing stem cell transplantation. Although protective isolation has demonstrated some efficacy in patients with acute leukemia, the cost is considerable, and the use of this approach is limited.

Prophylactic Antibiotics

Prophylactic antibiotics have demonstrated efficacy in reducing the risk of FN and documented infections. However, by definition, such prophylaxis must be broad spectrum and can be associated with toxicity, the emergence of antibiotic-resistant bacteria, and fungal overgrowth (2).

Trimethoprim-Sulfamethoxazole
- ❖ Trimethoprim-sulfamethoxazole clearly reduces the risk of *Pneumocystis carinii* pneumonia and may reduce the risk of bacterial infections.
- ❖ However, the lack of apparent effect on mortality and adverse reactions, including allergies to the sulfonamide, myelosuppression, and the development of drug resistant bacteria, as well as more frequent candidiasis have led the IDSA to recommend against routine prophylaxis with trimethoprim-sulfamethoxazole in neutropenic chemotherapy patients (2).

Quinolones
- ❖ The oral quinolones are used frequently for prophylaxis in neutropenic cancer patients. RCTs have demonstrated that the quinolone antibiotics are capable of preventing FN, infection, and reducing infection-related mortality in hematologic cancer patients receiving systemic chemotherapy.
- ❖ In a previous meta-analysis, reduction in the risk of gram-negative infection was observed but with no significant reduction in gram-positive infection, fungal infection, clinically documented infection, or infection-related deaths (25).
- ❖ A more recent meta-analysis reported a significant reduction, with fluoroquinolone prophylaxis, in all-cause as well as infection-related mortality, fever, clinically documented infections,

and microbiologically documented infections (26). All but three of the trials included entirely or mostly patients with hematologic malignancies with none of the solid tumor studies demonstrating significant reductions in mortality or infection-related mortality. Although the fluoroquinolones increase the risk of toxicity and resistant organisms after treatment, these differences were not statistically significant.

❖ Two additional trials of prophylactic fluoroquinolones have recently been reported in a mixture of patients with leukemia, lymphoma, and solid tumors (27,28). Significant reductions in the risk of FN, hospitalization for FN, and documented infections including bacteremia were observed with no significant difference in infection-related or overall mortality. The synchronous increase in resistant bacteria observed has again raised concern about the institutional and regional emergence of antibiotic resistance resulting from broad-scale use of antibiotic prophylaxis.

❖ The IDSA guidelines from 2002 recommend against routine FN prophylaxis with the fluoroquinolones (2). However, this represents an area of active investigation and bears close monitoring as recommendations may change. Although the quinolones are not approved by the U.S. Food and Drug Administration for use in children, it appears prudent to consider their use in infection prophylaxis in adults with acute leukemia and perhaps other high-risk populations. They should not be used in institutions in which parenteral quinolones are routinely used as part of empiric therapy or in which resistance has already been demonstrated.

Vancomycin

❖ Evidence for antibiotic resistance and limited clinical benefit argues against the use of prophylactic vancomycin in neutropenic patients (29).

Antifungal Prophylaxis

❖ Largely owing to the increasing frequency of fungal infections in patients with repeated episodes of FN, numerous studies of the potential benefit of prophylactic antifungal therapy have been conducted.

❖ RCTs of the azole antifungal agents including fluconazole have demonstrated reduction in the risk of fungal infections as well as fungal-related deaths in patients receiving systemic chemotherapy. The limited spectrum of fluconazole has led to recent studies of itraconazole. Meta-analyses of antifungal prophylaxis have demonstrated significant reductions in superficial and invasive fungal infection as well as fungal-related mortality (30,31). Most of the observed benefit was seen in studies of stem cell transplantation and hematologic malignancies. Invasive *Aspergillus* was not affected, except in subgroup analysis of the itraconazole studies (31). Concern remains that the prophylactic use of these agents may shift the fungal infection pattern to more dangerous azole-resistant species.

Prophylactic Colony-Stimulating Factors

❖ Crawford et al. (32) reported the first double-blind, placebo-controlled RCT of prophylactic granulocyte colony-stimulating factor (G-CSF) in adult patients receiving chemotherapy for small cell lung cancer demonstrating a reduction in the risk of FN and documented infection by approximately 50%.

❖ A meta-analysis of RCTs of prophylactic G-CSF confirmed the ability of prophylactic G-CSF to reduce the risk of FN and documented infection as well as to sustain dose intensity across a range of lymphoma and solid tumor populations and chemotherapy regimens (33). A significant increase in bone pain was observed in approximately 20% of patients.

❖ Similarly, a meta-analysis of prophylactic CSFs in childhood cancer patients has demonstrated a significant reduction in FN, documented infections, length of hospitalization, and use of amphotericin (34).

❖ A large, double-blind, placebo-controlled RCT of pegylated G-CSF (pegfilgrastim) in breast cancer patients demonstrated a reduction in risk of FN from 17% to 1% (35), consistent with previous studies suggesting a further reduction in risk of FN with pegfilgrastim compared to filgrastim (36,37).

❖ A previous economic analysis based on the Crawford trial and limited cost data suggested a FN risk threshold of 40%, at which the added cost of G-CSF is offset by the reduction of cost due to decreased hospitalization for FN (38). An updated economic analysis based on total direct hospital costs reported an FN threshold risk of approximately 20% (39).

❖ An updated meta-analysis of 14 RCTs of prophylactic G-CSF has demonstrated a significant reduction in risk of FN ($P < .0001$) and infection-related mortality ($P < .015$) while enabling delivery of greater chemotherapy-relative dose intensity (40).

❖ Recently published National Comprehensive Cancer Network (NCCN) Myeloid Growth Factor Guidelines recommend routine prophylaxis in cancer chemotherapy patients at a 20% or greater risk FN (6). The recommendations are based on recent RCTs and the updated cost data (41). The guidelines recommend an initial evaluation followed by an assessment of individual patient risk along with consideration of the treatment intention (Table 9). The risk assessment includes consideration of the treatment regimen and individual risk factors for the occurrence of FN (Figure 6), as well as those related to adverse medical consequences, including mortality, associated with FN (Table 7).

Table 9.   2005 National Comprehensive Cancer Network Guidelines: Primary Prophylaxis

	Treatment Intent		
Risk of FN[a]	Curative	Prolonged Survival/QALYs	Symptom Control/QOL
High (>20%)	CSF	CSF	CSF[b]
Intermediate (10%–20%)	Consider CSF	Consider CSF[a]	Consider CSF[b]
Low (<10%)	No CSF	No CSF	No CSF

CSF, colony-stimulating factor; FN, febrile neutropenia; QALYs, quality-adjusted life years; QOL, quality of life.
[a]Indicates risk of other neutropenic events compromising treatment efficacy.
[b]Alternative regimen or dose reduction and treatment delay may also be considered.
Modified from Crawford J, Althaus B, Armitage J, et al. Myeloid growth factors. J Natl Compr Canc Netw 2005;3:549–555.

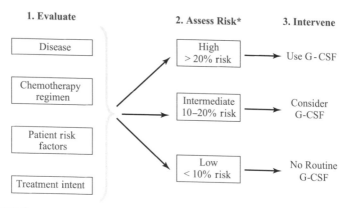

1. Evaluate   **2. Assess Risk***   **3. Intervene**

Figure 6
2005 National Comprehensive Cancer Network Guidelines for myeloid growth factor use in patients receiving cancer chemotherapy at risk for febrile neutropenia: decision tree for primary prophylaxis. *Risk of febrile neutropenia or neutropenic event compromising treatment. G-CSF, granulocyte colony-stimulating factor. (From Lyman GH. Guidelines of the National Comprehensive Cancer Network on the use of myeloid growth factors with cancer chemotherapy: a review of the evidence. J Natl Compr Canc Netw 2005;3:557–571, with permission.)

Summary and Conclusions

Myelosuppression and its complications, including FN, still represent the most important dose-limiting toxicity of systemic cancer chemotherapy, often compromising dose intensity in treatable and potentially curable malignancies. The development of FN represents a medical emergency requiring immediate evaluation and prompt administration of empiric broad-spectrum antibiotics. FN often occurs early in the course of chemotherapy and is not only associated with treatment intensity but also with factors related to disease and patient characteristics. Risk factors for serious medical complications, including mortality, have been identified and may assist in guiding the choice of therapy, including empiric antibiotics and myeloid growth factors. Nevertheless, FN continues to be associated with substantial morbidity, mortality, and cost. Therefore, considerable interest remains in efforts to prevent severe neutropenia and FN. Common sense dictates that diligent hygiene be used by health professionals to avoid the spread of infection among patients. Although effective in reducing the risk of FN and mortality in the hematologic malignancies, the role of prophylactic antibiotics in solid malignancies remains to be defined in the context of drug toxicity and emerging antibiotic resistance. The myeloid growth factors are indicated for prophylaxis of FN as well as sustaining or increasing chemotherapy dose intensity in the curative setting.

Acknowledgment

We would like to thank Connie French for her technical and administrative assistance in the preparation of this manuscript.

References

1. Common toxicity criteria for adverse events, Version 3, DCTD, NCI, NIH, DHHS. Available at: http://ctep.cancer.gov. Accessed March 31, 2003.
2. Infectious Diseases Society of America. 2002 Guidelines for the use of antimicrobial agents in neutropenic patients with cancer. Clin Infect Dis 2002;34:730–751.
3. Bodey GP, Buckley M, Sathe YS, et al. Quantitative relationships between circulating leukocytes and infection in patients with acute leukemia. Ann Intern Med 1966;64:328–340.
4. Dale D, McCarter GC, Crawford J, et al. Myelotoxicity and dose intensity of chemotherapy: reporting practices from randomized clinical trials. J Natl Compr Canc Netw 2003;1:440–454.
5. Lyman GH, Lyman CH, Agboola O. Risk models for predicting chemotherapy-induced neutropenia. Oncologist 2005;10:427–437.
6. Crawford J, Althaus B, Armitage J, et al. Myeloid growth factors. J Natl Compr Canc Netw 2005;3:549–555.
7. Lyman GH, Morrison VA, Dale DC, et al. for the ANC Study Group. Risk of febrile neutropenia among patients with intermediate-grade non-Hodgkin's lymphoma receiving CHOP chemotherapy. Leuk Lymphoma 2003;44:2069–2076.
8. Lyman GH, Delgado D. Risk and timing of hospitalization for febrile neutropenia in patients receiving CHOP, CHOP-R, or CNOP chemotherapy for intermediate-grade non-Hodgkin's lymphoma. Cancer 2003;98:2402–2409.
9. Levy MM, Fink MP, Marshall JC, et al. 2001 SCCM/ESICM/ACCP/ATS/SIS International Sepsis Definitions Conference. Crit Care Med 2003;31:1250–1256.

10. Schiel X, Hebart H, Kern WV, et al. Sepsis in neutropenia: Guidelines of the Infectious Diseases Working Party (AGIHO) of the German Society of Hematology and Oncology (DGHO). Ann Hematol 2003; 82(Suppl 2):S158–S166.

11. Wisplinghoff H, Seifert H, Wenzel RP, et al. Current trends in the epidemiology of nosocomial bloodstream infections in patients with hematological malignancies and solid neoplasms in hospitals in the United States. Clin Infect Dis 2003;36:1103–1110.

12. Gonzalez-Barca E, Fernandez-Sevilla A, Carratala J, et al. Prognostic factors influencing mortality in cancer patients with neutropenia and bacteremia. Eur J Clin Microbiol Infect Dis 1999;18:539–544.

13. Malik I, Hussain M, Yousuf H. Clinical characteristics and therapeutic outcome of patients with febrile neutropenia who present in shock: need for better strategies. J Infect 2001;42:120–125.

14. Darmon M, Azoulay E, Alberti C, et al. Impact of neutropenia duration on short-term mortality in neutropenic critically ill cancer patients. Intensive Care Med 2002;28:1775–1780.

15. Elting LS, Rubenstein EB, Rolston KV, et al. Outcomes of bacteremia in patients with cancer and neutropenia: observations from two decades of epidemiological and clinical trials. Clin Infect Dis 1997; 25:247–259.

16. Carratala J, Roson B, Fernandez-Sevilla A, et al. Bacteremic pneumonia in neutropenic patients with cancer: causes, empirical antibiotic therapy, and outcome. Arch Intern Med 1998;158:868–872.

17. Caggiano V, Weiss RV, Rickert TS, et al. Incidence, cost, and mortality of neutropenia hospitalization associated with chemotherapy. Cancer 2005;103:1916–1924.

18. Lyman GH, Dale D, Crawford J. Incidence, practice patterns, and predictors of low dose intensity in adjuvant breast cancer chemotherapy: Results of a nationwide study of community practices. J Clin Oncol 2003;21:4524–4531.

19. Lyman GH, Dale D, Friedberg J, et al. Incidence and predictors of low chemotherapy dose intensity in aggressive non-Hodgkin's lymphoma: A nationwide study. J Clin Oncol 2004:22:4302–4311.

20. Abeloff MD, Armitage JO, Niederhuber JE, et al., eds. Clinical oncology, 3rd ed. Philadelphia: Elsevier Churchill Livingstone, 2004.

21. Talcott JA, Siegel RD, Finberg R, et al. Risk assessment in cancer patients with fever and neutropenia: a prospective, two-center validation of a prediction rule. J Clin Oncol 1992;10:316–322.

22. Klastersky J, Paesmans M, Rubenstein EB, et al. The Multinational Association for Supportive Care in Cancer risk index: a multinational

scoring system for identifying low-risk febrile neutropenic cancer patients. J Clin Oncol 2000;18:3038–3051.

23. Ozer H, Armitage JO, Bennett CL, et al. 2000 Update of recommendations for the use of hematopoietic colony-stimulating factors: evidence-based clinical practice guidelines. J Clin Oncol 2000;18:3558–3585.

24. Clark OAC, Lyman GH, Castro AA, et al. Colony stimulating factors for chemotherapy induced febrile neutropenia: a meta-analysis of randomized controlled trials. J Clin Oncol 2005;23:4198–4214.

25. Engels EA, Lau J, Barza M. Efficacy of quinolone prophylaxis in neutropenic cancer patients: A meta-analysis. J Clin Oncol 1998;16: 1179–1187.

26. Gafter-Gvili A, Fraser A, Paul M, et al. Meta-analysis: Antibiotic prophylaxis reduces mortality in neutropenic patients. Ann Intern Med 2005;142:979–995.

27. Bucaneve G, Micozzi A, Menichetti F, et al. Levofloxacin to prevent bacterial infection in patients with cancer and neutropenia. N Engl J Med 2005;353:977–987.

28. Cullen M, Steven N, Billingham L, et al. Antibacterial prophylaxis after chemotherapy for solid tumors and lymphomas. N Engl J Med 2005;353:988–998.

29. Cruciani M, Malena M, Bosco O, et al. Reappraisal with meta-analysis of the addition of gram-positive prophylaxis to fluoroquinolone in neutropenic patients. J Clin Oncol 2003;21:4127–4137.

30. Bow EJ, Laverdiere M, Lussier N, et al. Antifungal prophylaxis for severely neutropenic chemotherapy recipients: a meta-analysis of randomized controlled trials. Cancer 2002;94:3230–3246.

31. Glasmacher A, Prentice A, Gorschlüter M, et al. Itraconazole prevents invasive fungal infections in neutropenic patients treated for hematologic malignancies: evidence from a meta-analysis of 3,597 patients. J Clin Oncol 2003;21:4615–4626.

32. Crawford J, Ozer H, Stoller R, et al. Reduction by granulocyte colony-stimulating factor of fever and neutropenia induced by chemotherapy in patients with small-cell lung cancer. N Engl J Med 1991;325:164–170.

33. Lyman GH, Kuderer NM, Djulbegovic B. Prophylactic granulocyte colony-stimulating factor in patients receiving dose intensive cancer chemotherapy: a meta-analysis. Am J Med 2002;112:406–411.

34. Sung L, Nathan PC, Lange B, et al. Prophylactic granulocyte colony-stimulating factor and granulocyte-macrophage colony-stimulating factor decrease febrile neutropenia after chemotherapy in children with cancer: a meta-analysis of randomized controlled trials. J Clin Oncol 2004;22:3350–3356.

35. Vogel CL, Lyman GH, Crawford J, et al. Predicting the risk of chemo-therapy-induced neutropenia in patients with breast cancer: rationale for prospective risk model development. Breast Cancer Res Treat 2002;76:S537.

36. Holmes FA, O'Shaughnessy JA, Vukelja S, et al. Blinded, randomized, multicenter study to evaluate single administration pegfilgrastim once per cycle versus daily filgrastim as an adjunct to chemotherapy in patients with high-risk Stage II or Stage III/IV breast cancer. J Clin Oncol 2002;20:727–731.

37. Green MD, Koelbl H, Baselga J, et al. A randomized double-blind multicenter phase III study of fixed-dose single-administration peg-filgrastim versus daily filgrastim in patients receiving myelosuppressive chemotherapy. Ann Oncol 2003;14:29–35.

38. Lyman GH, Lyman CG, Sanderson RA, et al. Decision analysis of hematopoietic growth factor use in patients receiving cancer chemo-therapy. J Natl Cancer Inst 1993;85:488–493.

39. Lyman GH, Kuderer N, Greene J, et al. The economics of febrile neu-tropenia: implications for the use of colony-stimulating factors. Eur J Cancer 1998;34:1857–1864.

40. Kuderer NM, Crawford J, Dale DC, et al. Meta-analysis of prophylac-tic granulocyte colony-stimulating factor (G-CSF) in cancer patients receiving chemotherapy. J Clin Oncol 2005;23:758s.

41. Lyman GH. Guidelines of the national comprehensive cancer network on the use of myeloid growth factors with cancer chemotherapy: a review of the evidence. J Natl Compr Canc Netw 2005;3:557–571.

42. Heussel CP, Kauczor HU, Heussel GE, et al. Pneumonia in febrile neu-tropenic patients and in bone marrow and blood stem-cell transplant recipients: use of high-resolution computed tomography. J Clin Oncol 1999;17(3):796–805.

Cancer Pain Management at the Bedside

Diane C. St. Germain, RN, MS, CRNP, and Ann Berger, MSN, MD

Pain is recognized as a very common symptom in individuals with cancer. In the general adult oncology population, the prevalence ranges from 18% to 100% with a mean of 40%. The prevalence increases with advanced cancer, ranging from 53% to 100%, with a mean of 74% (1). The cancer pain experience can be overwhelming, affecting the individual emotionally, spiritually, socially, and functionally. Furthermore, individuals with cancer often experience concomitant symptoms related to the cancer itself and/or treatment, including fatigue, diminished appetite, nausea, dyspnea, diarrhea/constipation, insomnia, and depression. Despite the impact pain has on quality of life and recognition of pain as a frequent and serious problem in individuals with cancer, the undertreatment of pain is pervasive. Barriers persist for health care professionals, the public, and patients with cancer and their families owing to inadequate priority, lack of education, and inappropriate attitudes (2). Inadequate assessment continues to be a problem that leads to poorly managed pain. There is discord between the physician's and the patient's report of pain, as demonstrated in a study done by Grossman et al. (3). It is no surprise that many individuals with cancer and their families fear that they will endure pain and suffering through the trajectory of their illness. This chapter provides an overview of pain in the individual with cancer, reviews pain assessment, and describes treatment approaches, including pharmacologic, interventional, and complementary approaches.

Etiology of Cancer Pain

Pain can occur in the setting of cancer through a variety of mechanisms. Most common, chronic cancer pain results from direct invasion of pain-sensitive structures by the tumor (4). In addition, individuals with cancer can experience pain due to diagnostic and therapeutic procedures, as well as cancer therapy (surgery, radiation, chemotherapy, immunotherapy). It is not uncommon for an individual to experience more than one etiology, which can intensify the pain experience.

Tumor Involvement (4,5)

- ❖ Invasion into cutaneous deep tissues and bone resulting in somatic pain
  - ◆ Bone pain
  - ◆ Muscle and soft tissue pain
  - ◆ Headache
- ❖ Injury to sympathetically innervated organs resulting in visceral pain
  - ◆ Hepatic distention syndrome
  - ◆ Midline retroperitoneal syndrome
  - ◆ Chronic intestinal obstruction
  - ◆ Peritoneal carcinomatosis
  - ◆ Malignant perineal pain
  - ◆ Adrenal pain syndrome
  - ◆ Ureteric obstruction
- ❖ Aberrant somatosensory processes caused by injury to nervous system resulting in neuropathic pain
  - ◆ Cranial neuralgias
  - ◆ Radiculopathies
  - ◆ Brachial plexopathy
  - ◆ Lumbosacral plexopathy
  - ◆ Peripheral mononeuropathies
  - ◆ Spinal cord compression

Diagnostic and Therapeutic Procedures (4,5)

- ❖ Lumbar puncture

- ❖ Needle biopsy
- ❖ Bone marrow biopsy
- ❖ Paracentesis/thoracentesis

Treatment Related (4,5)

- ❖ Surgical removal of tumor or metastases
  - ◆ Postoperative pain
  - ◆ Postmastectomy pain
  - ◆ Postradical neck dissection pain
  - ◆ Post-thoracotomy pain
  - ◆ Stump and phantom-limb pain
  - ◆ Lymphedema
- ❖ Chemotherapy
  - ◆ Mucositis
  - ◆ Peripheral neuropathy
  - ◆ Arthralgia and myalgia due to paclitaxel
  - ◆ Hand/foot syndrome (capecitabine)
  - ◆ Flare of bone pain with hormonal therapy for breast and prostate cancer
- ❖ Radiation therapy
  - ◆ Mucositis or esophagitis
  - ◆ Enteritis and proctitis
  - ◆ Myelitis
  - ◆ Chronic myelopathy
  - ◆ Plexopathy (brachial and lumbosacral)
  - ◆ Osteoradionecrosis
  - ◆ Skin "burns"
- ❖ Other
  - ◆ Growth factor–induced bone pain
  - ◆ Postherpetic neuralgia
  - ◆ Interleukin-2 and interferon-related myalgias

Pain Assessment

Poor assessment continues to be a chief cause of inadequately managed pain. This can lead to selection of an inappropriate medication for the type of pain experienced, inadequate dosing of an analgesic leading to poor pain relief, or excessive dosing leading to unpleasant side effects and limitation of available treatment modalities. In addition to an incomplete assessment is the failure to accept the patient's report of pain and the failure to act on the patient's report of the pain (6).

There are several pain assessment questionnaires that are useful in guiding the clinician toward a complete assessment (Table 1) (7).

Table 1.   Pain Assessment Questionnaires   .

Initial pain assessment tool

> The patient or nurse identifies the location of the pain by marking the figure drawings, then answers the following questions: intensity, quality, onset, duration, variations, rhythms, manner of expressing pain, what relieves pain, what causes or increases the pain, effects of pain on sleep, appetite, physical activity, relationship with others, emotions, concentration, and other.

Brief Pain Inventory

> Patients are asked to locate their pain on the figure drawings, rate their pain using an 11-point Likert scale (0–10) according to pain experienced in the last 24 h: worst, least, average, and right now. The patient then lists treatments or medications currently receiving for pain. The patient then rates on a Likert scale how much pain has interfered with mood, walking ability, work, relations with other people, sleep, and enjoyment of life over the past week.

Short-Form McGill Pain Questionnaire (SF-MPQ)

> Fifteen descriptors are rated on a 4-point severity scale; three scores are available, which reflect the sensory, affective, and total descriptors. The Present Pain Intensity index of the standard MPQ and a VAS are also included.

The Memorial Pain Assessment Card

> Consists of one verbal descriptor scale and three VAS scales measuring pain intensity, pain relief, and mood.

VAS, visual analog scale.
Adapted from McCaffery M, Pasero C. Assessment: underlying complexities, misconceptions, and practice tools. In: McCaffery M, Pasero C, eds. Pain: clinical manual. St. Louis: Mosby, 1999:35–102; and Anderson KO, Cleeland CS. The assessment of cancer pain. In: Bruera ED, Portenoy RK, eds. Cancer pain: assessment and management. New York: Cambridge Press, 2003:51–66.

In addition to a description of the pain experienced, some of the tools evoke information regarding the impact that pain has on quality of life. Beyond a description of the physical pain, assessment entails obtaining a thorough medical history, performing a physical examination, and obtaining appropriate diagnostic and laboratory studies, which will aid in determining the extent of malignant disease and causative factors contributing to the pain. Laboratory studies can identify liver or renal impairment, which may influence the analgesic and dosing used.

Additional Factors to Include in the Initial Pain Assessment

- ❖ Comorbidities
- ❖ Concurrent symptoms (fatigue, nausea, diarrhea/constipation, insomnia)
- ❖ Concurrent medications
- ❖ Psychosocial assessment
- ❖ Spiritual assessment
- ❖ Cultural influences and preferences
- ❖ Functional status
- ❖ Patient goals
- ❖ Family concerns and issues
- ❖ Patient-related barriers

Physical Pain Assessment

- ❖ Location
- ❖ Onset
- ❖ Duration
- ❖ Temporal pattern (continuous, intermittent)
- ❖ Characteristics of pain experienced (achy, cramping, burning)
- ❖ Intensity (at present, lowest, and highest level); see Table 2 (7)
- ❖ Acceptable or tolerable level of pain
- ❖ Aggravating factors
- ❖ Relieving factors
- ❖ Treatments tried, their effectiveness, and side effects experienced (include over-the-counter medications and alternative and complementary therapies)

Table 2. Pain Intensity Scales

Scale	Description	Advantages	Disadvantages
Verbal descriptor scale (VDS)	Patients are asked to describe their pain using the following descriptors: none, mild, moderate, severe, or excruciating. Pain relief is described in a similar way: none, slight, moderate, and complete.	Simple to use	There may be variable interpretation of the descriptors based on education, culture, or primary language spoken
Visual analog scale (VAS)	Patients are asked to rate the pain using a mark along a straight line with one end representing "no pain" and the opposite end representing "the worst pain experienced."	Easy to administer	May be difficult for some to comprehend Scoring can be time consuming
Numerical rating scale (NRS)	Patients are asked to rate the pain according to numbers along a horizontal line with "0" representing no pain and "10" representing the worst possible pain. Because cancer pain can vary, patients are often asked to rate the best, worst, and average level of pain they experienced over the past 24 h.	Often more easily understood than VDS or VAS The most commonly recommended scale in pain treatment guidelines Available in multiple languages Can be administered orally in very sick patients	May be difficult for some to comprehend
Faces rating scale (Oucher or Wong-Baker)	Pictures of faces depicting level of hurt from no pain (smiling face) to worst pain (sad, crying face) with correlated numeric ratings.	Can be used in pediatric population Translated into several languages	—

From Anderson KO, Cleeland CS. The assessment of cancer pain. In: Bruera ED, Portenoy RK, eds. Cancer pain: assessment and management. New York: Cambridge Press, 2003:51–66, with permission.

Psychosocial Assessment

- ❖ Current mood state
- ❖ History of psychiatric disorders
- ❖ Social support
- ❖ Financial stress and/or insurance issues
- ❖ Access to health care and/or medications
- ❖ Current use of illicit drugs and/or alcohol
- ❖ Past history of substance abuse
- ❖ Coping skills
- ❖ Home environment (physical layout, who is living in the home)
- ❖ Cultural considerations
- ❖ Primary language spoken, literacy
- ❖ Conflict within the family
- ❖ Loss and/or grief issues
- ❖ Fears

It is imperative that all of these factors are assessed during the initial pain assessment. An individual's mood state can influence the perception of pain as well as the patient's compliance with the treatment plan. When a patient is experiencing pain in the setting of depression or anxiety, the perception of the pain can be altered and often perceived as greater than in the absence of depression or anxiety. Furthermore, anxiety and depression can affect how the individual copes with the pain experience and the impact pain has on other aspects of their life (work, relationships, socially, and functionally).

In some situations, anxiety and/or depression overrides the pain experienced. An individual may cope with anxiety and/or depression by using opioids to treat their mood state. The individual may complain of persistent pain in the face of increased opioid dosing. Opioids may be taken to induce sedation to avoid dealing with the psychological issues at hand. Oftentimes, the clinician assessing the patient receives vague responses regarding the location, quality, and intensity of the pain experienced. The patient may be able to only express, "I hurt all over." If the patient is receiving patient-controlled analgesia (PCA), the record of bolus doses may reveal an unusually high number of attempted boluses compared to received boluses.

Addressing the psychological suffering issues with an antianxiety agent or an antidepressant coupled with counseling and emotional support leads to improved mood state, appropriate use of opioids for pain relief, and improved functional status. Additional interventions include the use of complementary modalities, such as massage, guided imagery, biofeedback, hypnosis, and Reiki therapy, all of which can aid in relaxation and focusing energy on the self.

In addition to assessing the psychological state, performing a spiritual assessment can provide additional information to manage the patient's pain and ability to cope. Beyond inquiring about the patient's religious preference, it is important to determine the meaning of being in pain for the patient. For some, being in pain holds value. Some believe it is necessary to be in pain as part of a punishment or feel they deserve to have cancer and pain because of poor judgments or actions of their past. Suffering is a large component for some religions. Patients may intentionally undertreat pain to endure suffering. Ambuel (8) developed a useful tool that uses the acronym *SPIRIT*. SPIRIT describes the patients overall spirituality, including his or her *s*piritual belief system, *p*ersonal spirituality, *i*ntegration with a spiritual community, *r*ituals practiced, *i*mplications for medical care, and *t*erminal events planning.

Spiritual History (8)

❖ Faith: Is spirituality a part of your life?
❖ Meaning: What meaning do you place on having this cancer pain? What is your meaning of being?
❖ Importance: What significance does your belief have on your disease?
❖ Community: Do you have a supportive spiritual community?
❖ Care: How can we attend to these spiritual needs in your care?

Another aspect of assessment is to determine the impact pain has on functional status. Altered function can be one of the most distressing effects of pain. Decreased function can effect the role the person has in his or her family. Is he or she the person that cooks, does housework, runs errands, cares for the children, drives children, or carries primary responsibility for the household income? For some, their career and work life is the essence of their being.

Functional Status Measurements

- ❖ Functional Living Index-Cancer
- ❖ Functional Assessment of Cancer Therapy (see Figure 1)

Patient-Related Barriers (9)

Last, identify patient-related barriers to the treatment of pain to complete a thorough pain assessment. Addressing these issues during the assessment phase can dispel myths, lessen fears, and obviate problems with successful pain management.

- ❖ Fear of addiction
- ❖ Fear of becoming tolerant to the effects of the medication
- ❖ Fear of side effects
- ❖ Belief that pain in cancer is inevitable and should be accepted
- ❖ "Good patients" should not complain about pain
- ❖ Complaints of pain would distract health care providers from curing the cancer
- ❖ Pain may be a sign of progressive disease
- ❖ Fear of injections

The barriers questionnaire developed by Ward et al. (10) has been widely used in studies to address the above-mentioned patient-related barriers. The questionnaire is a self-report instrument with 27 items and eight subscales outlining the eight barriers listed above. Each question is answered using a 6-point Likert-type scale. Gunnarsdottir et al. (9) updated the questionnaire and included the following items:

- ❖ Pain medications may impair immune function.
- ❖ Pain medications block or mask one's ability to monitor symptoms or changes in one's body.

Given these barriers, it is essential that patients and families receive education regarding opioid use to dispel myths and concerns. Health care providers should partner with patients to provide pain control and provide constant reassurance that the pain can be adequately managed.

When discussing barriers, it is important for patients and their families, as well as all health care providers involved in the care of

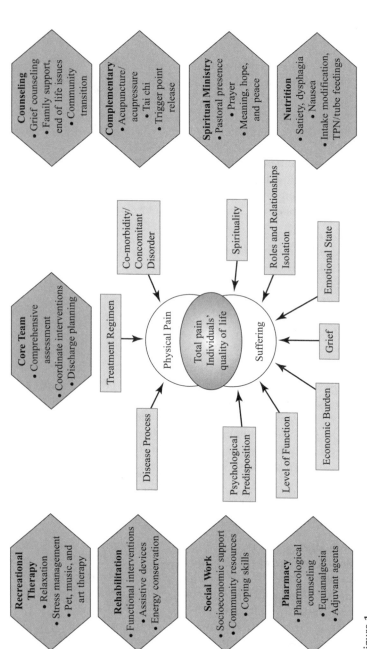

Figure 1

Nature of pain. TPN, total parenteral nutrition.

the patient, to understand the difference between tolerance, physical dependence, addiction, and pseudoaddiction. It is not uncommon for a patient to be labeled addicted or accused of abusing opioids based on a misunderstanding of these terms.

- ❖ *Tolerance*: the need to escalate doses of opioids despite a lack of change in the pain being treated. This is a rare occurrence, and, most likely, opioid doses require escalation because of worsening pain in the face of disease progression.
- ❖ *Physical dependence*: after approximately 1 week on steady dosing of opioids, the body becomes physically dependent on the medication. If one were to abruptly stop the opioids, withdrawal symptoms would occur. Hence, all opioids should be tapered over time. The experience of withdrawal can often be confused with addiction.
- ❖ *Addiction*: a psychological and behavioral process that encompasses three types of aberrant phenomenon: loss of control over drug use, compulsive drug use, and continued use despite harm. There is a craving for the opioid, and extreme measures will be taken to gain access (i.e., theft, prostitution, etc.). The risk involves those individuals who take opioids for reasons other than pain. The risk of addiction is very low in individuals who take opioids for pain.
- ❖ *Pseudoaddiction*: occurs when pain is being undertreated. The individual monitors very closely the timing of the opioids and is frequently asking for opioids more frequently than ordered and/ or for a higher dose. They are striving to get better pain control, not an inappropriate amount of opioids for other intentions.

Reassessment of Pain

The reassessment of pain is as critical as the initial assessment. The effectiveness of an opioid and its toxicity should be determined at the peak onset of action for the agent. For an oral agent, this should be done at 60 minutes, and, for an intravenous agent, this should be done at 15 minutes. Reassessment should also take place at the time trough and steady-state levels of the agent are reached. Reassessment should be done frequently in the cancer population not only to efficiently manage the individual's pain and monitor for side effects, but also because the pain can change over time. For individuals receiving cancer therapy, the pain may become less, necessitating a decrease in opioid dosing. Alternatively, the patient may experience progressive disease resulting in more intense pain, new sites of pain, or the onset of a new type of pain. Last, changes in the patient's other medical problems, medications, or psychosocial status can change the level of pain experienced by the patient, requiring a change in opioid dosing (Table 3) (2).

Treatment Approaches

All patients have the right to pain control. The hallmark of pain management is that the pain is being controlled in the setting of min-

Table 3.   Types of Pain

Type	Cause	Description	Examples	Treatment
Somatic	Nociceptor activation	Localized, aching, throbbing Gnawing feeling	Bone, joint pain	NSAIDs Opioids
Visceral	Nociceptor activation	Pressure, tightening, aching Pulling, stretching	Pleural, hepatic disease	Opioids NSAIDs Steroids
Neuro-pathic	Destruction of a nerve Peripherally or centrally	Severe, sharp, shooting, stabbing, burning, hot Numbness, tingling	Peripheral neuropathy Postherpetic neuralgia	Opioids Neuroleptics Tricyclic anti-depressants Steroids Acupuncture
Myofascial	Damage to the muscle	Tightness, pulling, spasm	Upper back, neck pain	NSAIDs Heat Stretching TENS Trigger point release

NSAIDs, nonsteroidal anti-inflammatory drugs; TENS, transcutaneous electrical nerve stimulation.

imal side effects and increased functioning. The approach is to start with the least invasive intervention and move to other interventions as the less invasive approaches become ineffective. The World Health Organization (WHO) developed an analgesic ladder, which provides a step-wise approach to the management of pain in accordance with the reported severity (mild, moderate, or severe). Analgesic therapy, according to the WHO ladder and anticancer treatment results in relief of pain for 70%–90% of patients (11).

❖ *Mild pain*: acetaminophen or nonsteroidal anti-inflammatory drugs (NSAIDs). Acetaminophen can be helpful for mild pain without an inflammatory component, such as headache or bone pain. The use of acetaminophen is limited to 4,000 mg/day. Persistent use at this level can lead to liver damage. NSAIDs are useful for mild pain as well as adjuvant therapy in the treatment of visceral, bone, and inflammatory pain.

❖ *Moderate pain*: opioids, such as codeine, hydrocodone, and oxycodone, all short-acting agents, administered on an as needed basis every 4–6 hours. Bear in mind, these opioids are often combined with acetaminophen, limiting the daily maximum amount. If the patient has constant pain, requires the opioid on a regular basis, or has severe pain, a long-acting opioid is warranted.

❖ *Moderate to severe pain*: opioids, such as morphine, oxycodone, hydromorphone, levorphanol, fentanyl, and methadone. All of these come in long-acting preparations or, in the case of methadone, have a long half-life and are used as a long-acting agent.

Guidelines for Initiating Opioid Therapy

I. Choose an opioid (see Table 4)
   A. Consider pain intensity
   B. Organ function
   C. Comorbidities
   D. Prior opioid use
   E. Available routes of administration and formulations (long acting vs. short acting)
   F. Availability
   G. Cost

Table 4. Types of Opioids

Mild-to-severe pain

    Short-acting oral preparations

        Codeine plus acetaminophen (Tylenol® with codeine, Ortho-McNeil)

        Hydrocodone plus acetaminophen or aspirin (Vicodin®, Abbott; Lortab®, UCB; Zydone®, Endo Labs; others)

        Oxycodone plus acetaminophen or aspirin (Percocet®, Endo Labs; Percodan®, Endo Labs; Tylox®, Ortho-McNeil; others)

        Tramadol (Ultram®, Ortho-McNeil)

Moderate-to-severe pain

    Short-acting preparations

        Oxycodone, immediate release (OxyIR®, Purdue Pharma; Roxicodone®, Elan)

        Morphine, immediate release

        Hydromorphone (Dilaudid®, Abbott)

        Oral transmucosal fentanyl citrate (Actiq®, Cephalon)

        Oxymorphone (in clinical development)

    Long-acting oral preparations

        Oxycodone, control release (OxyContin®, Purdue Pharma)

        Morphine, controlled release (MS Contin®, Purdue Frederick; Kadian®, Faulding Labs)

        Methadone (Dolophine®, Roxane; others)

        Fentanyl (Duragesic® patches, Janssen)

        Oxymorphone (in clinical development)

  II. Select route of administration
      A. Choose the least invasive route
      B. Consider patient compliance
      C. Available patient support (family to assist with administration if necessary)
 III. Dosing and dose titration
      A. Consider prior exposure to opioids and dosing requirement
      B. Dose according to pain intensity
      C. Perform ongoing reassessment and titrate to therapeutic effect or toxicity

D. Titrate upward by 25%–50%

E. Begin with as needed dosing to determine opioid requirement

F. Should frequent as needed dosing be required, pain is constant or severe, consider long-acting agent

G. Determine 24-hour opioid requirement and convert to long-acting agent

H. Provide short-acting agent for breakthrough dosing (5%–15% of long-acting opioid dose)

IV. Monitor and treat side effects

   A. Sedation

      1. May develop tolerance 2–3 days after initiation of an opioid or dose adjustment

      2. Assess use of other centrally acting agents

      3. Check organ function

      4. Adjust opioid dose by 30%–50%

      5. Sedation in setting of limited alternative therapies, consider a stimulant

   B. Nausea

      1. Consider other causative factors

      2. Assess bowel function

      3. Review concurrent medications

      4. Rotate opioids

      5. If other opioids not an option, medicate with an antiemetic

   C. Constipation

      1. Tolerance does not develop

      2. Prevent constipation with a daily bowel regimen

   D. Respiratory depression

      1. Monitor sedation in opioid-naïve patients

      2. Slow and safe titration

V. Opioid titration can be done after the first opioid has been titrated upward without adequate pain relief or the occurrence of intolerable side effects

Patient-Controlled Analgesia

During an acute pain crisis or postoperatively, PCA can be a very effective approach to achieve quick pain control. In addition, PCA can be useful when there is a need to efficiently determine the individual's opioid requirement. Last, it can be used if the individual is experiencing uncontrolled nausea and vomiting. PCA is contraindicated in persons with altered mental status.

Adjuvant Medications

Adjuvant medications are used to enhance analgesic effect, treat concurrent symptoms, and provide independent analgesia. See Tables 5 and 6 for a list of adjuvant medications.

Interventional Approaches

Pain relief can be achieved in 85%–95% of individuals using the WHO guidelines; however, in 5%–15% of the patients, alternative approaches should be considered. In situations where appropriate pharmacologic and complementary approaches have not resulted in adequate pain management or severe dose-limiting side effects are present, interventional or neurosurgical approaches can be used. Typically, they are used to supplement pharmacologic and complementary approaches (12).

Tables 7–9 (12,13) outline available interventional and neurosurgical approaches and their indications.

Complementary Approaches

The use of complementary therapies is becoming commonplace to supplement pharmacologic approaches to pain management. Individuals with cancer pain who have not achieved satisfactory relief of pain often seek complementary approaches on their own. However, there are more and more pain centers developing an integrative approach to pain management. The term *complementary* is often used interchangeably with alternative or unconventional. *Comple-*

Table 5. Neuropathic Agents

Drug Class/Agent	Analgesic Indication	Dosing	Special Considerations	Side Effects
Anticonvulsants				
Gabapentin	Postherpetic neuralgia Diabetic neuropathy Migraine headaches	300 mg TID Max 1,200 mg TID	Somnolence may require lower initial dosing Night-time dosing may facilitate sleep	Somnolence, diarrhea, mood swings, fatigue, nausea, dizziness
Carbamazepine	Trigeminal neuralgia Diabetic neuropathy	100–200 mg/day Max 1,200 mg/ day (DD)	Obtain CBC and LFTs before administration Monitor for agranulo- cytosis	Somnolence, dizziness, gait disturbance
Phenytoin	Trigeminal neuralgia	300 mg/day	Weak to moderate analgesic effect	Gingival hyperplasia, hirsutism
	Diabetic neuropathy	Max 15 mg/kg	Obtain CBC and LFTs before administration	
Valproic acid	Migraine, cluster and tension headaches	250 mg/day Max 1,000–2,000 mg/day (DD)	Multiple drug interac- tions	CNS depression, hepatic and hemato- logic toxicity
Lamotrigine	HIV neuropathy Trigeminal neuralgia Cold-induced allo- dynia	25–50 mg/day Max 200 mg BID, titrate slowly	For pain refractory to phenytoin and car- bamazepine Valproic acid ↓clear- ance	Rash, dizziness, ataxia, constipation, nausea, diplopia, somnolence

(continued)

Table 5. *Continued*

Drug Class/Agent	Analgesic Indication	Dosing	Special Considerations	Side Effects
Topiramate	Post-thoracotomy, RSD, headaches, intercostal neuralgia	25–50 mg/day Max 200 mg BID	Prolonged use may cause renal calculi Absorption slowed by food	Anorexia, weight loss
Oxcarbazepine	Trigeminal neuralgia	300–600 mg/day Max 2,400 mg/day	Similar to carbamazepine with less severe side effects	Skin sensitivity Hyponatremia
Tricyclic Antidepressants				
Desipramine (Norpramin®, Aventis)	Neuropathic and musculoskeletal pain	10–25 mg/bedtime Max 50–100 mg/bedtime	Less sedative and anticholinergic effects than amitriptyline	Dry mouth, sedation, cardiac arrhythmias, urinary retention
Amitriptyline (Elavil®, AstraZeneca)	Same	10–25 mg/bedtime Max 150 mg/bedtime	Take 10 h before planned waking to decrease side effects	Same
Nortriptyline (Pamelor®, Mallinckrodt)	Same	25 mg/bedtime Max 100–150 mg/bedtime		Same

Drug	Indication	Dose	Notes	Side effects
Benzodiazepines				
Clonazepam	Dysesthetic and paroxysmal pain	0.5–1.0 mg TID Max 20 mg/day (DD)	Long half-life, abrupt withdrawal could cause seizure Combine with anticonvulsant	Sedation, ataxia
Neuroleptic				
Olanzapine	Opioid-induced cognitive impairment	2.5–5.0 mg/day 20 mg/day	Safer neuroleptic, ↓extrapyramidal effects, ↓drug interactions, ↓neutropenia	Agitation, headache Insomnia somnolence
NMDA				
Methadone	Somatic and neuropathic pain	2.5 mg	May reduce opioid tolerance	
Ketamine	Refractory neuropathic pain	0.1–1.5 mg/kg/h	Poorly absorbed orally Do not use with ↑ICP, hypertension, psychosis	Confusion, hallucinations
Antiarrhythmics				
Mexiletine		50 mg TID Max 10 mg/kg/day	May worsen pre-existing cardiac arrhythmias, don't use in second and third degree AV blocks	Nausea, anxiety

(continued)

73

Table 5. *Continued*

Drug Class/Agent	Analgesic Indication	Dosing	Special Considerations	Side Effects
Lidocaine	Refractory neuropathic pain		Do not use with compromised cardiac contractility or conduction Avoid use of tricyclic antidepressants	
Anesthetics Systemic				
Mexiletine	Diabetic neuropathy	150 mg/day Max 900–1,200 mg/day	Monitor EKG at high doses Do not use in patient with arrhythmias	Nausea, dizziness
Local/cutaneous				
EMLA	Peripheral neuropathy, allodynia	Apply QID and cover with occlusive dressing		
Lidocaine (Lidoderm®, Endo Pharmaceuticals)	Postherpetic neuralgia			
Topical agents				
Capsaicin	Peripheral neuropathy	Apply QID		

Medication	Indication	Dose	Comments	Side effects
	Arthropathy			
	Mucositis			
Gelclair	Mucositis	Swish QID		
Corticosteroids				
Dexamethasone	Oncologic emergency (spinal cord or nerve compression); Refractory neuropathic pain; ↑ICP, organ distention, bone metastasis	80–100 mg IV ×1 then 10–12 mg IV QID; 4–16 mg PO (DD)	Improve pain, nausea, appetite, malaise; Longer duration of action (36–72 h); No mineralocorticoid effects (edema); Taper dosing to discontinue	Myopathy, delirium, depression
Prednisone		5–10 mg BID	Use to ↓myopathy; Taper dose to discontinue; Improve pain, nausea, appetite, malaise	Depression, delirium
α₂-Adrenergic agonist				
Clonidine	Diabetic neuropathy; Cancer-related neuropathy; Chronic headache	0.1 mg/day; 2 mg/day	Beneficial in less opioid-responsive patients; May reduce opioid requirement	Hypotension, dry mouth, somnolence

AV, atrioventricular; CBC, complete blood cell count; CNS, central nervous system; DD, divide doses; EKG, electrocardiogram; EMLA, eutectic mixture of local anesthetics; HIV, human immunodeficiency virus; ICP, intracranial pressure; LFT, liver function test; NMDA, N-methyl-D-aspartate; Max, maximum dose; RSD, reflex sympathetic dystrophy.

Table 6. Nonsteroidal Agents (NSAIDs)

Agent	Usual Starting Dose	Maximum Daily Dose	Comments
Aspirin	650 mg q4h PO	4,000 mg	Irreversibly inhibits platelet aggregation
Diflunisal (Dolobid®, Merck)	250–500 mg q8–12h PO	1,500 mg	Causes less gastric irritation compared to aspirin; increases acetaminophen level by 50% when coadministered
Choline magnesium tri-salicylate (Trilisate®, Purdue Frederick)	500–1,500 mg q12h PO	3,000 mg	Inexpensive; does not interfere with platelet aggregation
Diclofenac (Voltaren®, Novartis)	50–75 mg q8–12h PO	225 mg	Available in sustained release form
Etodolac (Lodine®, Ayerst)	200–400 mg q6–8h PO	1200 mg	Causes less gastric irritation especially in the elderly; antacids reduce peak concentration by 20%
Indomethacin (Indo-cin®, Merck)	25–50 mg q6–8h PO or rectally	200 mg	Associated with greater incidence and severity of toxicities
Sulindac (Clinoril®, Merck)	150–200 mg q12h PO	400 mg	Associated with less renal toxicity
Fenoprofen (Nalfon®, Mylan Pharmaceuti-cals)	300–600 mg q6h PO	3,200 mg	Associated with higher incidence of renal toxicity compared to other NSAIDs

Flurbiprofen (Ansaid®, Mylan Pharmaceuticals)	50–100 mg q6–8h PO	100 mg/dose; 300 mg/day	May cause CNS stimulation
Ibuprofen (Motrin®, McNeil Consumer)	200–800 mg q6–8h PO	3,200 mg	Associated with less gastric toxicity compared to other NSAIDs
Ketoprofen (Orudis®, Mylan Pharmaceuticals)	50–75 mg q6–8h PO	300 mg	Associated with higher incidence of dyspepsia compared to other NSAIDs; available in sustained release form
Naproxen (Naprosyn®, Roche Laboratories)	250–500 mg q8–12h PO	initial dose 1,250 mg/day, then 1,000 mg/day	May increase effects of phenytoin, warfarin, and sulfonylureas
Ketorolac (Toradol®, Roche Laboratories)	15–30 mg q6h IM or IV; 10 mg q4–6h PO	IM/IV, 120 mg; PO, 40 mg	Used only for pain (no antipyretic properties); only NSAID available in injectable form; not to be used for >5 days owing to potential toxicity
Meclofenamate (Meclomen®, Mylan)	50–100 mg q6h PO	400 mg	Rarely used owing to gastric and neurologic toxicities; associated with high incidence of diarrhea
Oxaprozin (Daypro®, Searle)	600–1,200 mg daily PO	1,800 mg	—

(continued)

Table 6. *Continued*

Agent	Usual Starting Dose	Maximum Daily Dose	Comments
Piroxicam (Feldene®, Pfizer)	10–20 mg daily PO	20 mg	Optimum efficacy may not occur for 1–2 wk; associated with high incidence of dyspepsia; increases the effect of phenytoin, warfarin, and sulfonylureas
Nabumetone (Relafen®, Glaxo-SmithKline)	1,000–2,000 mg daily PO; 500–750 mg two times per day	2,000 mg	Associated with high incidence of diarrhea
Celecoxib (Celebrex®, Pharmacia & Upjohn)	100–200 mg q12h PO	400 mg	Contraindicated if allergy to sulfa
Rofecoxib (Vioxx®, Merck)	12.5–25.0 mg daily PO	50 mg	No longer available because of increased cardiovascular problems
Meloxicam (Mobic®, Boehringer Ingelheim)	7.5–15.0 mg daily PO	15 mg	"Preferential" COX-2 activity; less selective than other COX-2 inhibitors

CNS, central nervous system; COX-2, cyclooxygenase-2; NSAIDs, nonsteroidal anti-inflammatory drugs.

Table 7. Interventional Approaches

Procedure	Description	Indication	Risks	Examples
Neurolytic procedures	Destruction of neurons that transmit pain	Pain limited to focal regions of the body. Used to target either peripheral nerves or centrally neuraxial (spinal cord or brain) nociceptors.	Pain can recur as well as worsen owing to architectural changes in the neuronal pathways. Nearby structures can be damaged. Risk of altered motor function, loss of bowel/bladder control.	Chemical neurolysis Uses chemical disruption of neuronal pathways conveying pain. Phenols in 5% glycerin or dehydrated ethanol are administered peripherally, epidurally, intrathecally, or to selective nerve roots. Cryoneurolysis Disrupts neuronal transmission by freezing tissue at the tip of the needle. Nerves in the region injected develop ice crystals resulting in lysis of axonal cell membranes. Continuous radiofrequency ablation A high-frequency voltage generator is used to produce localized heat to an active electrode, which is placed at the lesion to be treated.

From Mannes A, Lonser RR, Weil RJ, et al. Interventional and neurosurgical approaches for treating severe pain. In: Berger A, ed. Advances in cancer pain: a bedside approach. Chads Ford, PA: CMP Health Care Media, 2004:81–99, with permission.

Table 8. Interventional Procedures

Neurolytic Block	Procedure	Indication	Risk
Celiac plexus block	Can be achieved by an open surgical procedure (direct visualization), endoscopy, or percutaneous needle placement using radiographic imaging, which is the most common approach.	Pancreatic cancer, particularly involvement of the head of the pancreas versus the tail	Weakness (can be permanent), pneumothorax, hematuria, dissection of the aortic wall, transient hypotension, and diarrhea
Hypogastric plexus block	Can be done anteriorly or posteriorly using radiographic guidance. The needle is placed at L5-S1 vertebral junction and in the retroperitoneal space. A local anesthetic is injected to verify benefit and reduce pain that can be associated with ethanol injection.	Refractory pain due to tumors in pelvic area (vagina, uterus, cervix, testis, ovaries, and bladder)	Injury to the iliac vessels resulting in bleeding and hematoma formation, inadvertent IM or peritoneal injection
Intercostal nerve block	A short beveled needle is inserted between the ribs through the external and internal intercostal muscles to the intercostal space.	Chest wall pain due to disease, postsurgical scarring, nerve entrapment, or neuromas	Pneumothorax, hemothorax, hemoptysis, hematoma, intravascular injection, neuritis, subarachnoid block, infection
Vertebroplasty	Under guided radiologic imaging, one or two bone biopsy needles are inserted into the collapsed vertebral body through a small incision in the patient's back. Acrylic bone cement is injected to stabilize the fracture.	Pain associated with vertebral compression fractures due to metastatic tumors	Infection, pulmonary embolism from intravascular injection, weakness if the fracture is displaced or there is extravasation of the injection into the intrathecal space

From Mannes A, Lonser RR, Weil RJ, Tobias MD. Interventional and neurosurgical approaches for treating severe pain. In: Berger A, ed. Advances in cancer pain: a bedside approach. Chads Ford, PA: CMP Health Care Media, 2004:81–99, with permission.

Table 9. Neuraxial Medication Administration

Indication	Delivery Systems	Considerations

Uncontrollable pain
 	
Unacceptable side effects
 	
Need to use nonopioid analgesics
	Percutaneous catheter designed for short-term use (<1 wk); can have local reaction at insertion site and catheter has a tendency to migrate and dislodge
	
	An SC tunneled catheter prevents migration; appropriate for use in outpatient and home-bound patients
	
	Implanted catheter with SC injection site; placed in the epidural or intrathecal space; the SC injection port can be externalized or completely internalized
	
	Totally implanted catheter with implanted reservoir and manual pump currently in development and not yet commercially available
	
	Totally implanted catheter with implanted infusion pump
	
	  Constant fixed infusion pump—the dose can be adjusted by changing the concentration
	
	  Programmable infusion pump, which relies on cardiac pacemaker technology; through an external programmer head one can change the dose or give a single or continuous dose
		Patient life expectancy
		
		Costs
		
		Choice of epidural or intrathecal delivery route
		
		Duration of need

From Kim PS. Interventional cancer pain therapies. Semin Oncol 2005;32:194–199, with permission.

mentary therapy is used together with conventional medicine, as opposed to *alternative medicine*, which is used in place of conventional medicine. A variety of complementary therapies can augment pharmacologic approaches, lead to decreased opioid requirement, and address additional symptoms, such as anxiety, insomnia, nausea, and fatigue. Those using cognitive-behavioral techniques can decrease pain by altering pain transmission and pain perception by distracting the individual from the painful stimulus, inducing a relaxed state or altering mood or emotional context (14). Although not all-inclusive, the following outlines complementary approaches that are commonly used.

Rehabilitation Medicine Interventions

❖ *Massage*: the manipulation of muscle and connective tissue to promote their function and aid in relaxation and overall well-being.

❖ *Trigger point release*: myofascial trigger points are well-defined areas of tenderness or *knots* within a taut band of muscle. The use of needles with or without saline or anesthetic results in release of the knots with subsequent relief of pain. Stretch of the muscle often follows (15).

❖ *Transcutaneous electrical nerve stimulation*: high frequencies stimulate large-diameter myelinated afferent nerve fibers, which effect the pain messages within the spinothalamic tract by direct inhibition of an activated nerve or by activation of pain modulatory systems (15). Transcutaneous electrical nerve stimulation can be helpful for myofascial pain, muscle spasm, or chronic postsurgical neuropathic pain.

Other Interventions

❖ *Reflexology*: application of pressure to points on the body that are associated with specific glands or organs in the body. Reflexology releases tension, improves circulation, and promotes the body's natural functioning.

❖ *Reiki*: a Japanese word representing *universal life energy*. Reiki is a form of healing touch. By positioning their hands at the major chakras or energy centers of the body, the Reiki practitioner channels energy to replenish and rebalance the recipient's innate homeostatic mechanisms (16).

❖ *Therapeutic touch*: healing is promoted when the body's energies are in balance. The practitioner passes his or her hand over the patient and can identify energy imbalances. It is derived from an ancient technique called laying-on of hands (17).

❖ *Acupuncture*: uses the insertion of fine needles into the body at affected acupuncture points, which represent energy meridians by which *qi*, or life force or energy, flows. Insertion of the needles or firm pressure (*acupressure*) enhances the flow of qi, which improves ones state of health. It is thought that disease and/or symptoms ensue when the qi is out of balance.

Mind-Body Techniques

❖ Teach patients how to distance or distract themselves from the painful experience.

❖ *Relaxation techniques*: self-regulatory techniques that focus one's attention on a single word, thought, sound, prayer, sensation, or physical activity. Intrusive thoughts are eliminated with a return to the focus of one's attention (18).

❖ *Progressive muscle relaxation*: actively practices tensing and relaxing the 15 muscle groups throughout the body.

❖ *Guided imagery*: uses one's imagination to create mental images, using as many senses as possible (19).

❖ *Meditation*: a self-directed practice fostering nonjudgmental awareness of bodily sensations and mental activities. Relaxation occurs by clearing the mind with a single focus (i.e., a mantra) external focal point or internal focus, such as breathing. There are many forms of meditation including movement related, such as yoga, labyrinth walk, tai chi, and qi gong (18).

❖ *Hypnosis*: induces a state of selective, highly focused attention that is enhanced by imagery to heighten responsiveness to therapeutic suggestion (18).

❖ *Biofeedback*: the body's physiologic response to relaxation is recorded. This approach can be useful for individuals who benefit from seeing the effects of relaxation or feel the need to be in control during relaxation sessions.

In addition to the therapies, there are several other complementary modalities, previously listed, that may be helpful. These include prayer, music, art, and pet therapy.

Difficult Pain States

There are several challenging pain syndromes that occur frequently in the individual with cancer, necessitating interventions beyond opioid therapy. Although challenging, the pain can often be controlled with adjuvant medications and/or invasive procedures.

Neuropathic Pain

Neuropathic pain is related to a group of disorders that often results from injury to the central or peripheral nervous syndrome. Several etiologies contribute to the pain syndrome, including injury along the afferent and efferent pathways, tumor infiltration, chemotherapy, radiation, or surgery (20). Common surgical neuropathic pain is caused by the cutting of nerves during tumor resection, such as mastectomy, thoracotomy, and radical neck dissection. Radiation therapy can cause damage to the peripheral and central nervous systems, particularly after radiation to the brain or spinal cord. Chemotherapy, such as vincristine and paclitaxel, can cause peripheral neuropathy. Individuals experiencing neuropathic pain often describe burning, electrical, pinching, or shooting pain. In addition, they may describe a sensation of numbness, tingling, or "pins and needles." The pattern can be constant, intermittent, or episodic. Physical assessment may reveal paresthesias, dysesthesias, hyperalgesia, hyperpathia, or allodynia. See Table 5 for neuropathic agents.

Bone Pain

Bone metastases occur frequently in the setting of malignant disease, commonly in breast, lung, prostate, and kidney cancer and in multiple myeloma. Bone metastases affect the integrity of the bone and interfere with the normal processes of bone remodeling. Bone remodeling occurs in a setting in which there is a balance of osteoblast and osteoclast activity. Osteoblasts promote synthesis of new bone; osteoclasts play a role in bone resorption. Infiltration of tumor cells in the bone disrupts this process, resulting in an imbalance between bone development and bone destruction (21).

Pain associated with bone metastases is nociceptive somatic pain and can be associated with muscle and/or neuropathic pain. Somatic bone pain is often described as localized, constant throbbing, or aching. It is common for individuals to experience incident pain that occurs with movement or certain activities and then decreases at rest. Muscle spasms occur when the muscles surrounding bone lesions, particularly of the vertebral body, femur, and humerus, tighten to protect the weakened bone (22). Individuals experience grabbing or tightening of the area, particularly on movement. Last, neuropathic pain occurs when there is a compression or infiltration of nerves by the bone lesion (22). The pain is often described as intermittent, sharp, shooting, or lancinating. With nerve root involvement or spinal cord compression, individuals can experience burning, tingling, numbness, and radiation of pain along the distribution of the nerve. Refer to Table 6 for a list of nonsteroidal anti-inflammatory analgesics (NSAIDs).

Visceral Pain

Tumor invasion of an organ or viscera elicits a diffuse pain described as aching, colicky, cramping, pulling, or deep pressure. A tumor may involve organs of the gastrointestinal or genitourinary tracts, parenchymal organs, the peritoneum, or other retroperitoneal soft tissues.

Incident Pain

Incident pain is characterized by a sudden increase in pain associated with movement or other activities, such as coughing, swallowing, urination, or defecation. Typically, the pain subsides with inactivity. Incident pain is challenging to manage because by the time an opioid has reached its peak effect, the pain has subsided on its own through inactivity. Hence, dosing with opioids may result in sedation during the inactivity. However, certain movements or activities may be predictable, so the patient can be medicated before the inciting event. Oral transmucosal fentanyl can effectively be used for incident pain given its rapid onset and quick excretion.

Management of Pain in Challenging Patient Populations

The Elderly

The Agency for Health Care Policy and Research reported that the elderly are one of the most undertreated populations with regard to pain and should be considered a group at risk for mismanagement of pain and symptoms (23). This is attributed to the presence of inappropriate beliefs about pain sensitivity, pain tolerance, and use of opioids in the elderly. The elderly are often undertreated owing to multiple comorbidities, lack of assessment, and fear of medication side effects. In a landmark study of elderly patients with cancer pain, 29.4% of 13,625 patients ≥65 years old reported daily pain; of these patients, 25.5% received no analgesia (24). It is not uncommon to have the elderly receive psychoactive mediations when pain may be the root cause of behavioral symptoms.

Age can be an important variable affecting response to analgesia. Considerations should include the following (25):

1. Decline in organ function with increase in age, resulting in altered metabolism and elimination of drugs.
2. Changes in body composition, resulting in a decrease in the ratio of lean body mass to body weight with an increase in the proportion of body fat. Muscle and soft tissue mass and body water volume decrease.
   a. Lipid-soluble drugs (methadone, fentanyl) have a larger distribution and may have a delayed onset of action and accumulate.
   b. Water-soluble drugs (morphine, hydromorphone) have a lower volume of distribution, a higher peak, and slower decrease in plasma concentrations. The onset of action after a single dose of a hydrophilic opioid may be slightly faster and the duration of action slightly longer.
3. Decreased gastric motility and pH can affect absorption of NSAIDs, thereby increasing the risk of gastrointestinal bleeding and ulceration.

Patients with Current or Past History of Substance Abuse

Despite current or past history of substance abuse, adequate pain relief should remain the goal. Opioids should not be withheld, but rather given in a setting with the appropriate support. The following guidelines may be useful (26):

1. Accept and act on the patient's report of pain with appropriate assessment and treatment.
2. Reassure the patient of your commitment to providing pain relief.
3. Consult with an addiction specialist, and refer the patient to a drug rehabilitation center.
4. Consider involvement of a psychiatrist, particularly given the high incidence of depression in substance abuse.
5. Develop a written agreement and a copy of the treatment plan.
6. When opioid analgesics are necessary, use a long-acting agent, such as transdermal fentanyl or sustained-release morphine.

7. Provide clear instructions to the patient in writing.
8. Weekly visits.
9. Pill counts.
10. Random urine screens.
11. Prescribe a limited supply of opioids.

Refractory Pain at the End of Life

There remains a very small percentage of patients who experience severe, unrelenting pain at the end of life, despite appropriate pharmacologic and nonpharmacologic approaches. When this is the case, sedation may be considered.

According to Cherny (27), the justification of sedation in this setting is that it is goal appropriate and proportionate:

> At the end of life, when the overwhelming goal of care is the preservation of patient comfort, the provision of adequate relief of symptoms must be pursued even in the setting of a narrow therapeutic index for the necessary palliative treatments. In this context, sedation is a medically indicated and proportionate therapeutic response to the refractory symptoms, which cannot be otherwise relieved. Appeal to the patients' rights also underwrites the moral legitimacy of sedation in the management of otherwise intolerable pain at the end of life (27).

Conclusion

Pain is a very common symptom in individuals with cancer. It is recognized as a serious problem and for its impact on quality of life. Despite the available knowledge regarding pain management, many advances still need to take place to decrease the incidence of unrelieved pain. Performing a thorough assessment that considers physical, psychosocial, and spiritual needs, with frequent reassessment, and addressing clinician and patient barriers can provide a solid foundation toward successful pain management. We, as health professionals, may not always be able to cure the cancer or totally relieve the pain; however, we can help patients find meaning in their pain. The goal is to heal by helping the patient find a sense of wholeness in life.

References

1. Hearn J, Higginson IJ. Cancer pain epidemiology: a systematic review. In: Bruera ED, Portenoy RK, eds. Cancer pain: assessment and management. New York: Cambridge University Press, 2003: 19–37.
2. Levy MH, Samuel TA. Management of cancer pain. Semin Oncol 2005;32:179–193.
3. Grossman SA, Sheidler VR, Sweeden K, et al. Correlation of patient and caregiver ratings of cancer pain. J Pain Symptom Manage 1991;6:53–57.
4. Portenoy RK, Conn M. Cancer pain syndromes. In: Bruera ED, Portenoy RK, eds. Cancer pain: assessment and management. New York: Cambridge University Press, 2003:89–108.
5. McGuire DB. Occurrence of cancer pain. J Natl Cancer Inst Monogr 2004;32:51–56.
6. McCaffery M, Pasero C. Assessment: underlying complexities, misconceptions, and practice tools. In: McCaffery M, Pasero C, eds. Pain: clinical manual. St. Louis: Mosby, 1999:35–102.
7. Anderson KO, Cleeland CS. The assessment of cancer pain. In: Bruera ED, Portenoy RK, eds. Cancer pain: assessment and management. New York: Cambridge University Press, 2003:51–66.
8. Ambuel B. Taking a spiritual history #19. J Palliat Med 2003; 6(6):932–933.
9. Gunnarsdottir S, Donovan HS, Serlin RC, et al. Patient-related barriers to pain management: the barriers questionnaire II (BQ-II). Pain 2002;99:385–396.
10. Ward S, Goldberg N, Miller-McCauley V, et al. Patient-related barriers to management of cancer pain. Pain 1993;52:319–324.
11. World Health Organization. Cancer pain relief and palliative care. Report of a WHO expert committee. World Health Organization Technical Report Series, 804. Geneva: World Health Organization, 1990:1–75.

12. Mannes A, Lonser RR, Weil RJ, et al. Interventional and neurosurgical approaches for treating severe pain. In: Berger A, ed. Advances in cancer pain: a bedside approach. New York: CMP Healthcare Media, 2004:81–99.

13. Kim PS. Interventional cancer pain therapies. Semin Oncol 2005; 32:194–199.

14. Villemure C, Bushnell MC. Cognitive modulation of pain: how do attention and emotion influence pain processing. Pain 2002;92: 195–199.

15. Gillis TA. Rehabilitation medicine interventions. In: Bruera ED, Portenoy RK, eds. Cancer pain: assessment and management. New York: Cambridge University Press, 2003:238–260.

16. Thrapp L. Reiki. In: Herring, MA, Roberts MM, eds. Complementary and alternative medicine. Malden, Massachusetts: Blackwell Publishing, 2002:97–101.

17. What is complementary and alternative medicine (CAM)? National Center for Complementary and Alternative Medicine Web Site. Available at: http://nccam.nih.gov/health/whatiscam. Accessed September 2, 2005.

18. Handel D, Handel S. Nonpharmacological management of cancer pain. In: Berger A, ed. Advances in cancer pain: a bedside approach. New York: CMP Healthcare Media, 2004:101–117.

19. Kwekkeboom KL, Kneip J, Pearson L. A pilot study to predict success with guided imagery for cancer pain. Pain Manag Nurs 2003;4(3): 112–123.

20. Farrar JT, Portenoy R. Neuropathic cancer pain: the role of adjuvant analgesics. Oncology 2001;15:1435–1450.

21. Janjan N. Bone metastases: approaches to management. Semin Oncol 2001;28(Suppl 11):28–34.

22. Berger AM, Koprowski C. Bone pain: assessment and management. In: Berger AM, Portenoy RK, Weissman DE, eds. Principles and practice of palliative care and supportive oncology, 2nd ed. Philadelphia: Lippincott Williams & Wilkins, 2002:53–67.

23. Agency for Health Care Policy and Research. Clinical practice guideline: management of cancer pain. Rockville, Maryland: U.S. Department of Health and Human Services, 1994.

24. Bernabei R, Gambassi G, Lapane K, et al. Management of pain in elderly patients with cancer. JAMA 1998;279(23):1877–1882.

25. Pasero C, Reed BA, McCaffery M. Pain in the elderly. In: McCaffery M, Pasero C, eds. Pain: clinical manual. St. Louis: Mosby, 1999:674–710.

26. Compton P. Substance abuse. In: McCaffery M, Pasero C, eds. Pain: clinical manual. St. Louis: Mosby, 1999:428–466.

27. Cherny NI. The management of cancer pain. CA Cancer J Clin 2000;50(2):70–116.

Chemotherapy-Induced Nausea and Vomiting (CINV)

Wendy L. Wiser, DO, and Ann Berger, MSN, MD

Differential Diagnosis for Nausea and Vomiting

❖ Chemotherapy
❖ Opiates (morphine, codeine)
❖ Nonsteroidal anti-inflammatory drugs, erythromycin, aminophylline, digoxin, clonidine, etc.
❖ Infections (viral, bacterial)
❖ Increased intracranial pressure
❖ Head trauma
❖ Radiation therapy (total body radiation, abdominal radiotherapy)
❖ Peptic ulcer disease
❖ Anxiety, fear
❖ Vestibular or middle ear disease
❖ Bowel obstruction
❖ Constipation
❖ Metabolic disorders (uremia, hypercalcemia, hyponatremia, diabetic ketoacidosis, etc.)
❖ Severe pain

❖ Starting a new medication (e.g., selective serotonin reuptake inhibitor)
❖ Migraine headache
❖ Central nervous system neoplasms
❖ Withdrawal from substance abuse (drugs, alcohol)
❖ Carcinoma of the gastrointestinal tract
❖ Reye's syndrome
❖ Eye disorders (e.g., increased intraocular pressure)
❖ Abdominal trauma
❖ Conditioning (the sense memory of a significant episode of nausea and vomiting)
❖ Pregnancy
❖ Toxins and/or gastric irritants
❖ Psychiatric disorders (bulimia, anorexia nervosa)

Definition

Nausea is an unpleasant symptom associated with flushing, tachycardia, and the urge to vomit. *Vomiting* is the physical phenomenon that involves contraction of the abdominal muscles, descent of the diaphragm, and expulsion of stomach contents. Emesis is not always preceded by nausea, and, conversely, nausea does not necessarily result in vomiting. For some, feeling nauseous is much worse than vomiting owing to its lingering nature (1). Many physicians agree that nausea is more devastating than vomiting for a patient's quality of life (1–5).

Vomiting can be a self-protective mechanism if noxious substances are being expelled from the body; however, in the setting of chemotherapy, it is an unwanted and distressing response. Unfortunately, nausea and vomiting are ranked by patients as two of the most negative symptoms associated with receiving chemotherapy. Eight out of ten patients who receive chemotherapy experience nausea and vomiting (1,2). In spite of this fact, physicians still underestimate and suboptimally address the substantially disruptive nausea and emesis that are induced during the treatment of malignancy (1–6).

When we appreciate how much chemotherapy-induced nausea and vomiting (CINV) affects the overall care of our patients, we plan to prevent it with as much care and thought as when we choose the appropriate chemotherapies. The key to satisfactory management of CINV is prevention through pharmacologic and nonpharmacologic therapies before, during, and after chemotherapy.

Neurophysiology

The neural links that trigger nausea and vomiting are complex. A functional appreciation of the current theories about the emetic response involves a growing set of five main neurotransmitter groupings and seven noteworthy neural sites in the body.

Outside the blood–brain barrier (BBB) lies the chemoreceptor trigger zone, vestibular pathways, vagal afferents, and splanchnic nerves in the gastrointestinal tract; inside the BBB rests the higher cortical centers of the brain. These five oversimplified sources of input send data to the vomiting center (VC) for processing (7–14).

The main relay center for emetic response is at the VC, which is located inside the BBB in the neural networks of the lateral reticular formation of the medulla. The VC includes the areas of the medulla known as the dorsal motor nucleus of the vagus and the nucleus tractus solitarius. All sensory input is received and processed in the VC. It is here that afferent signals can be relayed into a vast vasomotor efferent cascade manifesting as nausea, retching, or emesis (7–14).

There are five main groupings of neurotransmitters identified as critical in this data exchange. An appreciation for their locations in the neural input cascade can be helpful in choosing an appropriate pharmacologic intervention for prevention and management of CINV (13).

The neurotransmitters discussed are serotonin type 3 (5-HT$_3$), dopamine type 3 (D3), muscarinic cholinergic, neurokinin type 1 (NK-1), and histamine type 1 (H1) (13,14). See Figure 1.

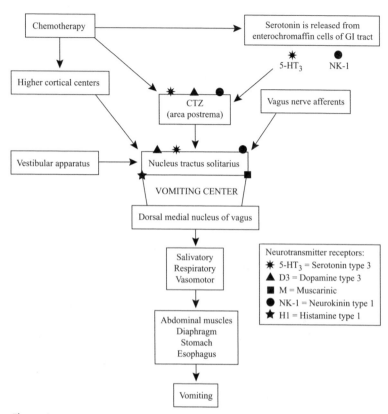

Figure 1
Neuronal pathways in chemotherapy-induced nausea and vomiting. CTZ, chemoreceptor trigger zone; GI, gastrointestinal. (From Dalal S, Bruera E. Pathophysiology of chemotherapy-induced nausea and vomiting, including emetic syndromes. In: Berger A, ed. Prevention of chemotherapy-induced nausea and vomiting. Manhasset, New York: CMP Healthcare Media, 2004:7.)

General Antiemetic Overview:
Neurotransmitter Receptor Antagonist

Receptor Blocked	Example	Medication Class Examples
Serotonin	5-HT$_3$	Ondansetron
		Granisetron
		Dolasetron
		Palonosetron
		Metoclopramide (at higher doses)
Dopamine	D3	Butyrophenones
		Haloperidol
		Droperidol
		Phenothiazines
		Chlorpromazine
		Prochlorperazine
		Thiethylperazine
		Metoclopramide
Neurokinin	NK-1	Aprepitant
Unknown	—	Steroids
		Dexamethasone
Muscarinic	Ach-m	Scopolamine
		Glycopyrrolate
Histamine	H1	Meclizine
		Cyclizine
		Diphenhydramine

Ach-m, muscarinic-subtype acetylcholine.

Classifications

CINV has traditionally been classified into three main categories (acute, delayed, and anticipatory) with two other related subtypes (breakthrough and refractory). These categories are based on the time of onset and pattern of occurrence in relation to the time of chemotherapy administration (8).

Chemotherapy-Induced Nausea and Vomiting Types at a Glance

Type	Timing (15)	Recommendations	
		Pharmacologic	Nonpharmacologic
Acute	Up to 24 h after chemotherapy (16)	$5\text{-}HT_3$ antagonist NK-1 antagonist Steroid Lorazepam Metoclopramide	Consider acupressure wrist bands; acupuncture, guided imagery; hypnosis
Delayed	24 h post-chemotherapy; may last 6–7 days (17) Often follows uncontrolled acute CINV	NK-1 antagonist $5\text{-}HT_3$ antagonist Steroid Lorazepam Metoclopramide	Same as above
Anticipatory	Consequence of CINV with initial chemotherapy; occurs before subsequent chemotherapy (18)	Optimal antiemetic therapy based on guidelines at every cycle, as appropriate	Strongly consider nonpharmacologic adjuncts (e.g., hypnosis, music therapy, etc.)
Break-through	CINV despite preventative steps Requires rescue medications	Same as above; plus at least one additional agent from a different class at the lowest effective dose	Same as above
Refractory	Symptoms that occur despite rescue medications	Same as above	Same as above

Evaluation

Experience has shown that there are known risk factors that increase the likelihood of a person to have nausea and vomiting related to receiving chemotherapy. There are patient-specific risk factors as well as chemotherapy-associated risk factors.

When choosing a chemotherapeutic regimen for the patient, it would be helpful to have historical patient information to assess his or her personal risk for developing CINV. Coupled with the clinician's appreciation for the inherent emetogenicity of the chemotherapy itself, this knowledge helps protect the patient from nausea and emesis.

Risk Factors for CINV

Patient Specific	Chemotherapy Specific
Female	Drug emetogenicity risk level (1–5) (see Risk for Emesis with Commonly Used Chemotherapy Drugs, later)
Age >6 yr, <50 yr	
<100 g ethanol intake/day for several years	
	Previous episode of CINV
Tendency for motion sickness	Higher doses
History of hyperemesis with pregnancy	Multiple doses
Tendency for anxiety	Multiple chemotherapy agents

From Osoba D, Zee B, Pater J, et al. Determinants of postchemotherapy nausea and vomiting in patients with cancer. J Clin Oncol 1997;15:116–123, with permission.

During the course of chemotherapy, nausea and/or vomiting may occur. When assessing nausea and vomiting, assess them separately. It is important to appreciate whether the patient's nausea is linked to emesis.

Consider the following questions during the evaluation:

❖ What is the timing, severity, duration, and mitigating factors associated with the nausea and/or vomiting?

❖ What does the emesis look like or contain?

❖ When was the last bowel movement?

❖ What medications has the patient had recently to mitigate the nausea and/or vomiting?

❖ What was the patient's past experience with chemotherapy (if any)?

❖ What are the patient's specific risk factors for having developed CINV? (See Risk Factors for CINV, earlier.)

❖ What were the chemotherapy-specific risk factors that are contributing to the CINV? (See Risk Factors for CINV, earlier, and the next section.)

Risk for Emesis with Commonly Used Chemotherapy Drugs[a]

Risk Level	Frequency of Emesis (%)	Drug (Dose)
5 (High)	>90	Carmustine (>250 mg/m^2)
		Cisplatin
		Cyclophosphamide ($1,500$ mg/m^2)
		Dacarbazine (>500 mg/m^2)
		Mechlorethamine
		Streptozocin
		Dactinomycin
		Pentostatin
		Lomustine (>60 mg/m^2)
4/3 (Moderate)	>30–90	Cyclophosphamide ($<1,500$ mg/m^2 PO)
		Carmustine (<250 mg/m^2)
		Doxorubicin
		Cisplatin (<50 mg/m^2)
		Epirubicin
		Cytarabine (>1 g/m^2)
		Idarubicin
		Hexamethylmelamine (PO)
		Ifosfamide
		Carboplatin
		Irinotecan
		Melphalan
		Procarbazine
		Mitoxantrone (>12 mg/m^2)
		Cytarabine (>1 g/m^2)

Risk for Emesis with Commonly Used Chemotherapy Drugs[a]   *Continued*

Risk Level	Frequency of Emesis (%)	Drug (Dose)
2 (Low)	10–30	Methotrexate (>100 mg/m^2)
		Fluorouracil (<1 mg/m^2)
		Doxorubicin (<20 mg/m^2)
		Mitoxantrone (<12 mg/m^2)
		Cytarabine (<1 mg/m^2)
		Temozolomide
		Etoposide (PO)
		Asparaginase
		Gemcitabine
		Mitomycin
		Paclitaxel
		Thiotepa
		Topotecan
		Docetaxel
		Aldesleukin (interleukin-2)
1 (Minimal)	<10	Capecitabine
		Vincristine
		Vinblastine
		Vinorelbine (IV)
		Teniposide (IV)
		Etoposide (IV)
		Bleomycin
		Rituximab
		Trastuzumab
		Methotrexate (<100 mg/m^2)

[a]In the absence of prophylactic antiemetic treatment.
Original table based on NCCN Antiemesis Practice Guidelines Panel. Antiemesis clinical practice guidelines. Oncology 2004;19(5):642; and adapted from Ettinger DS, Foran J, eds. New recommended guidelines for the treatment of CINV. NCCN 2004 Antiemetic Guidelines Review. Guidelines in Focus. 2004.

Management

It is important that the clinician is aware of pharmacologic and non-pharmacologic measures for prevention and management of CINV.

Pharmacologic Agents

Antiemetics As a Whole

In general, the mechanism of antiemetics is to block one or more neurotransmitter receptors in the complex cascade linked to the VC in the brain.

The information in the following general antiemetic dosing chart includes general information about antiemetics as well as specific recommendations for prevention and treatment of CINV.

General Antiemetic Groups

- ❖ Serotonin antagonists
- ❖ Dopamine antagonists
- ❖ NK-1 antagonists
- ❖ Steroids
- ❖ Adjunct medications (e.g., anticholinergics, antihistamines, cannabinoids, octreotide)
- ❖ Benzodiazepines

General Antiemetic Dosing Chart

Medication	Suggested Dose (Route)	Side Effects	Comments
Serotonin antagonists (1)			
Ondansetron	8 mg IV or 0.15 mg/kg IV q3h ×3 12–24 mg PO qd or 8 mg PO BID	Mild headache Constipation Lightheadedness Diarrhea Mild sedation Asymptomatic liver Transaminase Elevation Rarely EPS	First dose 30 min before chemo-therapy; no renal adjustment

General Antiemetic Dosing Chart   *Continued*

Medication	Suggested Dose (Route)	Side Effects	Comments
Granisetron	2 mg PO qd or 1 mg PO q12h 0.01 mg/kg IV over 5 min (1 mg IV max dose qd)	See above Taste changes	PO first dose <1 h before chemother-apy; IV first dose <30 min before chemotherapy; no renal adjustment
Dolasetron	100 mg PO or IV 1.8 mg/kg IV	See above	See above
Palonosetron (19)	No oral form, 0.25 mg IV	Headache Constipation QT prolongation	Give 30 min before chemotherapy; 40-h half-life; no renal adjustment
Dopamine antagonists (1)			
Metoclopra-mide	5–20 mg PO/IV q6h 4–8 mg PO BID	EPS (greater risk if younger)	Pretreat with diphenhydramine to decrease EPS when using to pre-vent/treat CINV; prolonged half-life with renal failure; >10-mg dose should be given IVPB; avoid in bowel obstruction
Chlorprom-azine	10–25 mg PO q4h 25–50 mg IV/IM q4h 50–100 mg PR q6h	Sedation Tardive dyskine-sia Hypotension NMS	May use for intrac-table hiccups
Haloperidol	0.5–5.0 mg PO, SC, IV q8h (max 100 mg in 24 h)	NMS EPS Tardive dyskinesia Drowsiness Anticholinergic effects Gynecomastia	Half-life approxi-mately 20 h; usual max 30 mg/day

(continued)

General Antiemetic Dosing Chart   *Continued*

Medication	Suggested Dose (Route)	Side Effects	Comments
Prochlorpera-zine	5–10 mg PO/IM q6h 2.5–10.0 mg IV q3h 25 mg PR BID	Drowsiness NMS, tardive dyskinesia; dry mouth, consti-pation, urinary retention	Multiple adverse reaction risks; max 40 mg/day
Neurokinin antagonists (20)			
Aprepitant	See specific CINV preven-tion and treat-ment guidelines	Diarrhea Fatigue Hiccups Constipation Rarely neutropenia	Contraindicated with cisapride and pimozide (for QT prolon-gation risk)
Steroid (1)			
Dexametha-sone	4–8 mg PO BID 8–20 mg IV qd 0.5–0.6 mg/kg DIV q12h	Mood swings Insomnia Peptic ulcer Appetite increase	Increase dose as needed; often dosed empirically
Methylpred-nisolone	125 mg IV	See above	Used as a substitute for dexametha-sone in CINV prevention and treatment
Antihistamine			
Diphenhy-dramine	25–50 mg PO q4h 10–50 mg IV q2h	Drowsiness Dry mouth Urinary retention Confusion	Max 400 mg/day; EPS treatment dose is 50 mg
Hydroxyzine	25–100 mg PO/IM q6h	See above Bitter taste Headache	Max 600 mg/day
Meclizine	25–50 mg PO q2h	Drowsiness Dry mouth Confusion Nausea and vomiting Tachycardia	

General Antiemetic Dosing Chart   *Continued*

Medication	Suggested Dose (Route)	Side Effects	Comments
Anticholinergic			
Scopolamine	1.5 mg patch q72h 0.6–1.0 mg IV/ SC q4h	Dry mouth Blurred vision Urinary retention Tachycardia	In palliative care, used for excess secretions and with intestinal obstruction
Glycopyrro- late	1–2 mg PO BID; 0.1–0.2 mg IM/IV q6h	Constipation Dry mouth Urinary retention Tachycardia	Same as above
Cannabinoid			
Dronabinol	2.5–5.0 mg PO q6h (max 20 mg/day)	Dysphoria Somnolence Difficulty concen- trating	Generally better tolerated in younger patients
Benzodiazepine			
Lorazepam	0.5–2.0 mg PO, SL, IV q6h	Sedation Amnesia	Not intrinsically an antiemetic; very useful as an adjunct; see CINV Guidelines (20)
Miscellaneous			
Octreotide	50–300 mcg SC BID (max 1,500 mcg/ day)	Diarrhea Dizziness Biliary tract abnormal Fatigue Fever	Start at 50 mcg and titrate up based on response; used in palliative med- icine for nausea and vomiting due to complete bowel obstruc- tion; decreases secretions

EPS, extrapyramidal side effects; NMS, neuroleptic malignant syndrome.
Note: These dosing guidelines are not meant to replace U.S. Food and Drug Administration guidelines or clinical judgment.

Antiemetic Use for Prevention and Treatment of Chemotherapy-Induced Nausea and Vomiting

Dynamic and evolving antiemetic guidelines have been constructed based on levels of clinical experience for prevention and treatment of CINV based on emetogenicity of the chemotherapeutic agent. Patients receiving moderate- to high-risk chemotherapy (levels 3, 4, and 5) should be protected from nausea and vomiting for at least 4 days.

Additional guidelines for those who experience breakthrough nausea and vomiting and those who are receiving radiation therapy are included in the next section.

General CINV Prevention and Treatment Guidelines Based on Level of Emetogenic Risk

Chemotherapy Risk	Antiemetic	Day 1	Day 2	Day 3	Day 4
High	Aprepitant	X	X	X	—
	Dexamethasone	X	X	X	X
	5-HT$_3$ antagonist	X	X	X	X
	Lorazepam	X	X	X	X
Moderate	Dexamethasone	X	X	X	X
		and	or	or	or
	5-HT$_3$ antagonist	(Palo)	X	X	X
		and	or	or	or
	Lorazepam	X	X	X	X
		Consider	or	or	
	Aprepitant	X	X	X	—

Palo, palonosetron preferred Day 1; X, medication recommended; —, none recommended to be given.
Original table based on NCCN Antiemesis Practice Guidelines Panel. Antiemesis clinical practice guidelines. Oncology 2004;19(5):642; and adapted from Ettinger DS, Foran J, eds. New recommended guidelines for the treatment of CINV. NCCN 2004 Antiemetic Guidelines Review. Guidelines in Focus. 2004.

Treatment Guidelines for Anticipatory, Breakthrough, and Refractory Chemotherapy-Induced Nausea and Vomiting

Anticipatory Emesis

❖ Prevention of CINV with optimal antiemetic treatment at every cycle of chemotherapy and/or radiation therapy
❖ Strongly consider nonpharmacologic modalities/adjuncts
❖ Alprazolam, 0.5–2.0 mg orally four times a day
❖ Lorazepam, 0.5–2.0 mg orally on the night before and morning of treatment (20)

Breakthrough and Refractory Chemotherapy-Induced Nausea and Vomiting

❖ Strongly consider additional nonpharmacologic measures.
❖ If nausea or vomiting persists, then add another agent at lowest efficacious dose from a different class [for specific dosing guidelines refer to NCCN Guidelines 2004 (20)].
❖ List of possible options depending on clinical scenario are as follows:
  ◆ Prochlorperazine
  ◆ Thiethylperazine
  ◆ Metoclopramide
  ◆ Lorazepam
  ◆ Ondansetron
  ◆ Granisetron
  ◆ Dolasetron
  ◆ Haloperidol
  ◆ Dronabinol
  ◆ Dexamethasone (20)

Treatment Guidelines for Prevention of Radiation-Induced Nausea and Vomiting with and without Chemotherapy

❖ Recommendation depends on type of radiation, dose, and location to the body (radiation therapy to upper abdomen and total body radiation are associated with greater nausea and vomiting).

❖ The recommended antiemetics (ondansetron, dexamethasone, or granisetron) are to be given pretreatment for each day of radiation therapy.

❖ For radiation therapy in combination with chemotherapy, refer to recommendations based on emetogenic potential of the chemotherapy (20).

Specific Antiemetic Doses for Chemotherapy-Induced Nausea and Vomiting Based on the Level of Emetogenic Risk

I. CINV prevention guidelines for highly emetogenic drugs (days 1–4)

II. CINV prevention guidelines for moderately emetogenic drugs (days 1–4)

III. CINV prevention guidelines for low emetogenic drugs

IV. CINV prevention guidelines for minimally emetogenic drugs

I. Chemotherapy-Induced Nausea and Vomiting Prevention Guidelines for Highly (Level 5) Emetogenic Drugs

Notes

❖ The order of the medications is not meant to indicate preference.

❖ Use lowest efficacious dose.

❖ Be mindful of potential side effects.

❖ Day 1 medications are to be given prechemotherapy.

❖ When fractionated doses of level 3–5 chemotherapy are given or there is a high risk of delayed CINV, daily dexamethasone, daily 5-HT_3 (or a one-time dose of palonosetron for 3-day chemotherapy regimen), and daily aprepitant (up to 3–5 days) should be given.

Medication	Dose (Route)
Day 1	
NK-1	Aprepitant, 125 mg PO qd
and	
Steroid	Dexamethasone, 12 mg PO or IV qd
	or
	Methylprednisolone, 125 mg IV qd
and	
5-HT$_3$ antagonist	Palonosetron, 0.25 mg IV qd (recommended on day 1; owing to long half-life, no follow-up dose necessary)
	or
	Ondansetron, 16–24 mg PO qd
	or
	Ondansetron, 8 mg (max 32 mg) IV
	or
	Granisetron, 2 mg PO qd or 1 mg PO BID
	or
	Granisetron, 0.01 mg/kg (max 1 mg) IV qd
	or
	Dolasetron, 100 mg PO qd
	or
	Dolasetron, 1.8 mg/kg IV qd or 100 mg IV qd
and	
Benzodiazepines	Lorazepam, 0.5–2.0 mg PO, IV, or SL q6h scheduled
Days 2–4	
NK-1	Aprepitant, 80 mg PO qd (day 2 and day 3)
and	
Steroid	Dexamethasone, 8 mg PO or IV qd
	or
	Methylprednisolone, 125 mg IV qd

(continued)

Continued

Medication	Dose (Route)
or	
5-HT$_3$ antagonist	Ondansetron, 8 mg PO or IV qd
	or
	Granisetron, 2 mg PO qd or 1 mg PO BID
	or
	Granisetron, 0.01 mg/kg (max 1 mg) IV qd
	or
	Dolasetron, 100 mg PO qd
	or
	Dolasetron, 1.8 mg/kg IV qd or 100 mg IV qd
and	
Benzodiazepines	Lorazepam, 0.5–2.0 mg PO, IV or SL q6h scheduled

Original table based on NCCN Antiemesis Practice Guidelines Panel. Antiemesis clinical practice guidelines. Oncology 2004;19(5):642; and adapted from Ettinger DS, Foran J, eds. New recommended guidelines for the treatment of CINV. NCCN 2004 Antiemetic Guidelines Review. Guidelines in Focus. 2004.

II. Chemotherapy-Induced Nausea and Vomiting Prevention Guidelines for Moderately (Levels 3–4) Emetogenic Drugs

Notes

❖ The order of the medications is not meant to indicate preference.
❖ Use lowest efficacious dose.
❖ Be mindful of potential side effects.
❖ Day 1 medications are to be given prechemotherapy.
❖ When fractionated doses of levels 3–5 chemotherapy are given or there is a high risk of delayed CINV, daily dexamethasone, daily 5-HT$_3$ (or a one-time dose of palonosetron for 3-day chemotherapy regimen), and daily aprepitant (up to 3–5 days) should be given.

Medication	Dose (Route)
Day 1	
Steroid	Dexamethasone, 12 mg PO or IV qd
	or
	Methylprednisolone, 125 mg IV qd
and	
5-HT$_3$ antagonist	Palonosetron, 0.25 mg IV (preferred on Day 1; owing to long half-life, no follow-up dose necessary)
	or
	Ondansetron, 16–24 mg PO
	or
	Ondansetron, 8 mg (max 32 mg) IV qd
	or
	Granisetron, 1–2 mg PO or 1 mg PO BID
	or
	Granisetron, 0.01 mg/kg (max 1 mg) IV qd
	or
	Dolasetron, 100 mg PO
	or
	Dolasetron, 1.8 mg/kg IV or 100 mg IV qd
and	
Benzodiazepines	Lorazepam, 0.5–2.0 mg PO, IV, or SL; PO q6h scheduled
and maybe	
NK-1	Aprepitant, 125 mg PO, if using carboplatin, cyclophosphamide, doxorubicin, epirubicin, ifosfamide, irinotecan, or methotrexate
Days 2–4	
Steroid	Dexamethasone, 8 mg PO or IV qd
	or
	Dexamethasone, 4 mg PO BID
	or
	Methylprednisolone, 125 mg IV qd

(continued)

Continued

Medication	Dose (Route)
or	
5-HT$_3$ antagonist	Ondansetron, 8 mg PO BID or 16 mg PO qd
	or
	Ondansetron, 8 mg (max 32 mg) IV qd
	or
	Granisetron, 1–2 mg PO qd or 1 mg PO BID
	or
	Granisetron, 0.01 mg/kg (max 1 mg) IV qd
	or
	Dolasetron, 100 mg PO qd
	or
	Dolasetron, 1.8 mg/kg IV or 100 mg IV qd
	or
	Metoclopramide, 0.5 mg/kg PO or IV q6h scheduled ± diphenhydramine, 25–50 mg PO or IV q4–6h prn
	or
	Metoclopramide, 20 mg PO q6h scheduled ± diphenhydramine, 25–50 mg PO or IV q4–6h prn
or	
NK-1	Aprepitant, 80 mg PO (continued on days 2–3, started day 1)
	and
	Dexamethasone, 8 mg PO or IV qd
	±
Benzodiazepines	Lorazepam, 0.5–2.0 mg PO, IV, or SL q6h scheduled

Original table based on NCCN Antiemesis Practice Guidelines Panel. Antiemesis clinical practice guidelines. Oncology 2004;19(5):642; and adapted from Ettinger DS, Foran J, eds. New recommended guidelines for the treatment of CINV. NCCN 2004 Antiemetic Guidelines Review. Guidelines in Focus. 2004.

III. Chemotherapy-Induced Nausea and Vomiting Prevention Guidelines for Low (Level 2) Emetogenic Drugs

Medication	Dose	Adjuvant Medication
Dexamethasone	12 mg PO/IV qd	± Lorazepam, 0.5–1.0 mg PO, IV, or SL q4–6h scheduled
or		
Prochlorperazine	10 mg PO or IV q4–6h scheduled	
or		
Prochlorperazine	15 mg spansule PO q8–12h scheduled	
or		
Thiethylperazine	10 mg PO q4–6h scheduled	
or		
Metoclopramide	20–40 mg PO q4–6h scheduled or 1–2 mg/kg q3h scheduled ± Diphenhydramine 25–50 mg PO or IV q4h scheduled ± Lorazepam 0.5–2.0 mg PO or IV q6h scheduled	

Original table based on NCCN Antiemesis Practice Guidelines Panel. Antiemesis clinical practice guidelines. Oncology 2004;19(5):642; and adapted from Ettinger DS, Foran J, eds. New recommended guidelines for the treatment of CINV. NCCN 2004 Antiemetic Guidelines Review. Guidelines in Focus. 2004.

IV. Chemotherapy-Induced Nausea and Vomiting Prevention Guidelines for Minimally (Level 1) Emetogenic Drugs

❖ Use agents listed under Chemotherapy-Induced Nausea and Vomiting Prevention Guidelines for Low (Level 2) Emetogenic Drugs prophylactically prechemotherapy and in the first 24 hours of level 1 emetogenic drug therapy.

Specific Dose Recommendations for Treatment of Breakthrough and Delayed Chemotherapy-Induced Nausea and Vomiting

Notes

- ❖ Consider scheduling antiemetic for a few doses until the symptoms show marked improvement.
- ❖ Give additional medication(s) from at least one different class when faced with breakthrough CINV.

Medication	Dose (Route)
Prochlorperazine	25 mg PR q12h
	or
	10 mg PO or IV q4–6h scheduled
	or
	15-mg spansule PO q8–12h scheduled
or	
Thiethylperazine	10 mg PR or PO q4–6h scheduled
or	
Metoclopramide	20–40 mg PO q4–6h scheduled
	or
	1–2 mg/kg q3–4h scheduled
	± Diphenhydramine, 25–50 mg PO or IV q4–6h scheduled
or	
Lorazepam	0.5–2.0 mg PO q4–6h scheduled
or	
Ondansetron	8 mg PO or IV qd
or	
Granisetron	1–2 mg PO qd or 1 mg PO BID
	or
	0.01 mg/kg (max 1 mg) IV qd

Continued

Medication	Dose (Route)
or	
Dolasetron	100 mg PO qd
	or
	1.8 mg/kg IV or 100 mg IV qd
or	
Haloperidol	1–2 mg PO q4–6h scheduled
	or
	1–3 mg IV q4–6h scheduled
or	
Dronabinol	5–10 mg PO q3–6h scheduled
or	
Dexamethasone	12 mg PO or IV (if not previously given) qd
or	
Methylprednisolone (Solu-Medrol®, Pharmacia & Upjohn)	125 mg IV qd

Original table based on NCCN Antiemesis Practice Guidelines Panel. Antiemesis clinical practice guidelines. Oncology 2004;19(5):642; and adapted from Ettinger DS, Foran J, eds. New recommended guidelines for the treatment of CINV. NCCN 2004 Antiemetic Guidelines Review. Guidelines in Focus. 2004.

Specific Dose for Prevention and Treatment for Anticipatory Chemotherapy-Induced Nausea and Vomiting

Medication	Dose (Route)
Alprazolam	0.5–2.0 mg PO q6h scheduled
Lorazepam	0.5–2.0 mg PO HS prechemotherapy and the AM pretreatment

Original table based on NCCN Antiemesis Practice Guidelines Panel. Antiemesis clinical practice guidelines. Oncology 2004;19(5):642; and adapted from Ettinger DS, Foran J, eds. New recommended guidelines for the treatment of CINV. NCCN 2004 Antiemetic Guidelines Review. Guidelines in Focus. 2004.

Nonpharmacologic Measures

In addition to standardized pharmacologic approaches to prevention and management of CINV, now, more than ever, patients have access to a multitude of nonpharmacologic therapeutic options. The specific mechanism of action of these interventions is not understood. The possibilities of intervention at the various complex levels of input to the VC are compelling (21–27).

Nonpharmacologic Therapy Considerations for Prevention and Treatment of Chemotherapy-Induced Nausea and Vomiting

- ❖ Acupressure
- ❖ Acupuncture
- ❖ Hypnosis
- ❖ Meditation and/or prayer
- ❖ Relaxation
- ❖ Biofeedback
- ❖ Imagery
- ❖ Distraction
- ❖ Music therapy
- ❖ Aromatherapy
- ❖ Herbals
- ❖ Therapeutic touch
- ❖ Reiki therapy

Clinical Pearls

1. CINV is regulated by the central nervous system.
2. The most satisfactory management of CINV is prevention.
3. Choose antiemetic therapy at the same time as chemotherapy choice.
4. Choose antiemetic therapy based on patient risk factors, planned chemotherapy agent and dose, and chemotherapy regimen schedule.

5. Patients receiving chemotherapy with higher risk for emesis (levels 3, 4, and 5) need antiemetics for at least 4 days.
6. Patients receiving chemotherapy for many days are at risk for acute and delayed CINV.
7. Patients with breakthrough CINV need antiemetic coverage from at least two different classes.
8. Choose an antiemetic, being mindful of possible side effects and toxicities.
9. Use the lowest effective dose of chosen antiemetic(s) before chemotherapy or radiation therapy.
10. When breakthrough or refractory nausea continues, consider the different potential mechanisms—central, vestibular, gastrointestinal—and treat with the appropriate medications.
11. Vestibular nausea is commonly seen in patients with motion sickness or hyperemesis during pregnancy and is best treated with meclizine, scopolamine patch, and acupressure point stimulation (MH-6).

References

1. Berger AM, Clark-Snow RA. Nausea and vomiting. In: DeVita VT Jr., Hellman S, Rosenberg SA, eds. Cancer: principles & practice of oncology, 7th ed. Lippincott Williams & Wilkins, 2005:2515–2522.
2. Lindley CM, Hirsch JD, O'Neill CV, et al. Quality of life consequences of chemotherapy-induced emesis. Qual Life Res 1992;1:331–340.
3. Osoba D, Zee B, Warr D, et al. Effect of postchemotherapy nausea and vomiting on health-related quality of life. The Quality of Life and Symptom Control Committees of the National Cancer Institute of Canada Clinical Trials Group. Support Care Cancer 1997;5:307–313.
4. Osoba D, Zee B, Warr D, et al. Quality of life studies in chemotherapy-induced emesis. Oncology 1996;53(Suppl 1):92–95.
5. Rusthoven JJ, Osoba D, Butts CA, et al. The impact of postchemotherapy nausea and vomiting on quality of life after moderately emetogenic chemotherapy. Support Care Cancer. 1998,6:389–395.
6. Fromer M. Chemotherapy-induced nausea and vomiting: research update on improving control. Oncology Times 2005;Jan 10:29–33.
7. Ossi M, Anderson E, Freeman A. 5-HT$_3$ receptor antagonists in the control of cisplatin-induced delayed emesis. Oncology 1996;53:78–85.

8. Borison HL, Wang SC. Physiology and pharmacology of vomiting. Pharmacol Rev 1953;5:193–230.

9. Carpenter DO. Neural mechanisms of emesis. Can J Physiol Pharmacol 1990;68:230–236.

10. Miller AD, Wilson VJ. "Vomiting center" reanalyzed: an electrical stimulation study. Brain Res 1983;270:154–158.

11. Wang SC. Emetic and antiemetic drugs. In: Root WS, Hofmann FG, eds. Physiological pharmacology: a comprehensive treatise, Vol. II. New York: Academic Press, 1965:255–328.

12. Dienmunsch P, Grelot L. Potential of substance P antagonists as antiemetics. Drugs 2000;60:533–546.

13. Leslie RA, Shah Y, Thejomayen M, et al. The neuropharmacology of emesis: the role of receptors in neuromodulation of nausea and vomiting. Can J Physiol Pharmacol 1990;68:279–288.

14. Wamsley JK, Lewis MS. Autoradiographic localization of muscarinic cholinergic receptors in rat brainstem. J Neurosci 1981;1:176–191.

15. ASHP. ASHP therapeutic guidelines on the pharmacologic management of nausea and vomiting in adult and pediatric patients receiving chemotherapy or radiation therapy or undergoing surgery. Am J Health Syst Pharm 1999;56:729–764.

16. Hesketh PJ, Kris MG, Grunberg SM, et al. Proposal for classifying the acute emetogenicity of cancer chemotherapy. J Clin Oncol 1997; 15:103–109.

17. Yalcin S, Tekuzman G. Serotonin receptor antagonists in prophylaxis of acute and delayed emesis induced by moderately emetogenic, single-day chemotherapy: a randomized study. Am J Clin Oncol 1999; 22:94–96.

18. Andrykowski MA, Jacobsen PB. Prevalence, predictors, and course of anticipatory nausea in women receiving adjuvant chemotherapy for breast cancer. Cancer 1988;62:2607–2613.

19. Aloxi™. Palonosetron HCL injection package insert. Minneapolis: MGI Pharma, Inc., 2003.

20. Ettinger DS, Foran J, eds. New recommended guidelines for the treatment of CINV. NCCN 2004 Antiemetic Guidelines Review. Guidelines in Focus. 2004.

21. Handel D. Role of nonpharmacologic techniques. In: Berger A, ed. Prevention of chemotherapy-induced nausea and vomiting. Manhasset, New York: CMP Health Care Media, 2004:91–110.

22. King CR. Nonpharmacologic management of chemotherapy-induced nausea and vomiting. Oncol Nurs Forum 1997;24(7):41–48.

23. Burish TG, Snyder SL, Jenkins RA. Preparing patients for cancer che-motherapy: affect of coping preparation and relaxation interventions. J Consult Clin Psychol 1991;59(4):518–525.
24. Roscoe JA, Morrow GR, Hickok JT, et al. The efficacy of acupressure and acustimulation wrist bands for the relief of chemotherapy-induced nausea and vomiting. A University of Rochester Cancer Center Community Clinical Oncology Program multicenter study. J Pain Symptom Manage 2003;26:731–742.
25. Roscoe JA, Morrow GR, Bushunow P, et al. Acustimulation wrist-bands for the relief of chemotherapy-induced nausea. Altern Ther Health Med 2002;8:56–63.
26. Butkovic D, Toljan S, Matolic M, et al. Comparison of laser acupuncture and metoclopramide in postoperative nausea and vomiting prevention in children. Paediatr Anaesth 2005;15(1):37–40.
27. Thompson A. Role of other antiemetics. In: Berger A, ed. Prevention of chemotherapy-induced nausea and vomiting. Manhasset, New York: CMP Health Care Media, 2004:57–89.

Constipation and Diarrhea

Joyson Karakunnel, MD, and Apurva A. Modi, MD

Constipation

Constipation is an extremely common symptom in the U.S. population as a whole, with prevalence rates as high as 28%. The prevalence in advanced cancer patients and in those who are receiving cancer treatment is 55% and 50%, respectively (1). For oncology patients, it is a major cause of costly hospital admissions. Hence, appropriate prevention and treatment guidelines are imperative to improve quality of life in a cost-effective manner.

Definition

Constipation can be defined by the presence of two or more criteria (Rome II criteria) listed below (2). The criteria should be present for at least 12 weeks within the last year but do not have to present consecutively. There should also be an absence of loose stools and insufficient criteria for diagnosing irritable bowel syndrome (IBS).

- ❖ Straining in at least 25% of defecations
- ❖ Feeling of incomplete evacuation in at least 25% of defecations
- ❖ Hard or lumpy stools on at least 25% of defecations
- ❖ Sensation of anorectal obstruction/blockade in at least 25% of defecations

❖ Use of manual maneuvers (e.g., digital evacuation) in at least 25% of defecations
❖ Frequency of stools of less than three per week

Etiology

Constipation can be classified as primary, secondary, or iatrogenic:

❖ Primary causes
  ♦ Inadequate fluid intake owing to chronic debilitating illnesses, and in oncologic patients secondary to nausea, weakness, or depression
  ♦ Low-fiber diet
  ♦ Lack of activity due to surgery, dramatic weight loss, or lethargy
❖ Secondary causes
  ♦ The secondary causes can be broadly classified into obstructive lesions of the gastrointestinal tract and neurogenic, metabolic, and endocrine abnormalities (Table 1).
❖ Iatrogenic causes
  ♦ Iatrogenic constipation results from the use of pharmacologic agents, chemotherapeutic drugs, and medical intervention. This is probably the most common cause of constipation in individuals with cancer. The drugs commonly involved are listed in Table 2.

Pathophysiology

Constipation can be classified into normal transit constipation, pelvic floor dysfunction, and slow transit constipation. In the largest series of 1,000 patients with intractable constipation, 59% had normal colonic transit, 28% had pelvic floor dysfunction, and 13% had slow colonic transit (3).

Normal Transit Constipation

❖ Normal rate of stool movement through the colon with normal frequency.

Table 1.   Secondary Causes of Constipation

Obstructive	Neurogenic
Strictures	Autonomic neuropathy
Colon cancer	Diabetes mellitus
Anal fissure	Chagas' disease
Proctitis	Hirschsprung's disease
Postsurgical lesions	Multiple sclerosis
Endocrine	Spinal cord injury
Hypothyroidism	Parkinson's disease
Panhypopituitarism	Others
Metabolic	Systemic sclerosis
Hypercalcemia	Amyloidosis
Hypokalemia	Anorexia nervosa
Hypomagnesemia	Pregnancy
Uremia	Depression
	Immobility

❖ Patients may have increased stress factors and, hence, perceive problems with constipation (4).

❖ Symptoms respond to treatment with dietary fiber and/or osmotic laxatives (5).

Pelvic Floor Dysfunction

❖ Synonyms include anismus, outlet obstruction, obstructed defecation, pelvic floor dyssynergia, dyschezia, and paradoxic pelvic floor contraction.

❖ Normal or slightly slowed colonic transit with extended periods of stool storage in the rectum (3,6).

❖ Symptoms include feeling of anal blockage, severe straining, prolonged defecation, and manual disimpaction.

❖ Inability to evacuate contents from the rectum may be secondary to loss of coordination between the abdominal, recto-anal, and pelvic floor muscles during defecation (7).

❖ Other mechanisms proposed are incomplete relaxation or paradoxic contraction of the pelvic floor muscles and external anal sphincter during defecation (6).

Table 2. Drugs Associated with Constipation

Over-the-counter medications
  Nonsteroidal anti-inflammatory drugs
  Antacids (calcium and aluminum containing)
  Calcium supplements
  Iron supplements
  Antidiarrheal medications

Prescription medications
  Opiates
  Anticholinergics
    Antidepressants
    Antispasmodics
    Antipsychotics
  Antiparkinsonian drugs
  Calcium channel blockers
  Diuretics
  Antihistamines
  Vinca alkaloids

Adapted from Locke GR 3rd, Pemberton JH, Phillips SF. AGA technical review on constipation. American Gastroenterological Association. Gastroenterology 2000;119:1766–1778.

Slow Transit Constipation

❖ Slow rate of stool transit through the colon and the rectum.
❖ In patients with minimal delay, dietary and cultural factors may play a role, and this can be reversed with a high-fiber diet.
❖ In patients with more severe slow-transit constipation, two subtypes have been identified:
  ◆ Colonic inertia—It is associated with no increase in motor activity after meals or after the administration of bisacodyl (8), cholinergic agents, or anticholinesterases (9). This is related to dysfunction and alterations in the enteric nerve plexus neurons expressing the excitatory neurotransmitter substance P (10) as well as a decrease in the number of Cajal's interstitial cells (11), which regulate gastrointestinal motility.

◆ Uncoordinated motor activity in the distal colon that acts as a functional barrier to normal transit (12).

Clinical Evaluation

The evaluation of a patient with constipation includes a thorough history and physical examination.

History

❖ Detailed drug history with emphasis on the use of opioids, anticholinergics, and calcium channel blockers.
❖ Family history significant for inflammatory bowel disease or colon cancer.
❖ Questions about symptoms associated with systemic diseases that cause constipation.
❖ Frequency, consistency of stools, and amount of straining associated with defecation; excessive straining could suggest other associated symptoms, such as abdominal pain, bloating, early satiety, weight loss, or rectal bleeding.
❖ Amount of straining associated with defecation; excessive and prolonged straining along with the need for perineal or vaginal pressure or digital evacuation could suggest slow transit constipation.
❖ Symptoms of alternating diarrhea and constipation with abdominal pain, bloating, and malaise that occurs between bowel movements could suggest IBS (13).
❖ The severity of symptoms can be graded using the National Cancer Institute Common Criteria for Adverse Events (Table 3).
❖ Weight loss, anorexia, malaise, and blood in stools could suggest a malignant process, such as colon cancer.
❖ Frequency, dosage, and type of laxatives, suppositories, or enemas used to relieve constipation.

Physical Examination

❖ Inspect the perianal region for tumors, external hemorrhoids, scars, fistulas, fissures, or fecal soiling. The anal reflex can be tested by a scratch test.

Table 3.   National Cancer Institute Common Terminology Criteria for Adverse Events in Constipation

Grade	Symptoms	Treatment
1	Occasional	Occasional use of stool softeners, laxatives, or enemas
2	Persistent	Frequent use of laxatives or enemas
3	Interfering with activities of daily living	Manual evacuation
4	Hemodynamic instability	—
5	Death	—

Adapted from de Roy van Zuidewijn DB, Schillings PH, Wobbes T, et al. Morphometric analysis of the effects of antineoplastic drugs on mucosa of normal ileum and ileal anastomoses in rats. Exp Mol Pathol 1992;56:96–107.

❖ Observe the descent of the perineum by asking the patient to bear down. Reduced descent (normal is between 1.0 and 3.5 cm) may indicate pelvic floor dysfunction, and increased descent may indicate laxity of the perineal muscles (e.g., after multiple pregnancies), which may lead to incomplete evacuation (14).

❖ Observe for prolapse of anorectal mucosa during the act of straining.

❖ Digital rectal examination:

◆ Examine for tumors, strictures, internal hemorrhoids, or fecal impaction.

◆ Evaluate the anal sphincter tone. A patulous opening may raise the suspicion for a neurologic disorder or trauma as the cause of constipation.

◆ Palpate the posterior border of the rectum formed by the puborectalis muscle. Tenderness along this border suggests puborectalis spasm syndrome.

◆ Ask the patient to simulate the act of defecation with the examiner's finger in place to test coordination of the pelvic muscles responsible for defecation.

◆ Test a sample of the stool for occult blood.

❖ Examine for rectocele, and consider a gynecologic consultation.

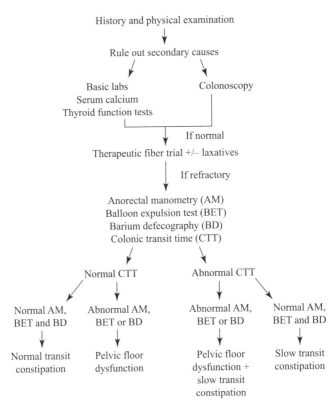

Figure 1
Diagnostic algorithm for constipation. (Adapted from Locke GR 3rd, Pemberton JH, Phillips SF. American Gastroenterological Association medical position statement: guidelines on constipation. Gastroenterology 2000;119:1761.)

Diagnostic Tests

Initial workup of a patient with constipation should include tests to rule out secondary causes (Figure 1). The laboratory tests of importance are as follows:

- ❖ Serum electrolytes and calcium
- ❖ Blood glucose
- ❖ Thyroid function tests
- ❖ Complete blood count

❖ Endoscopy: Colonoscopy is useful to detect lesions, which occlude the bowel like polyps, strictures, or tumor
❖ Barium enema is useful for detecting obstructive lesions of the colon and diagnosing megacolon and megarectum, as well as demonstrating proximal dilatation of the aganglionic colonic segment in Hirschsprung's disease

Once the secondary causes have been ruled out, further tests to determine the cause of constipation can be performed:

❖ Colonic transit time testing
  ◆ Transit time testing is performed by making the patient swallow radio-opaque markers in a gelatin capsule and taking abdominal radiographs 120 hours later (15).
  ◆ Prolonged transit is indicated by the retention of ≥20% of the markers. (Normal colonic transit time is 72 hours.)
❖ Defecography
  ◆ Defecography is performed by introducing thickened barium into the patient's rectum. Evacuation of the barium is observed by radiographic films or videos taken during fluoroscopy with the patient sitting on a specially constructed radiolucent commode (16).
  ◆ It helps to detect the following:
    • Anorectal angle during defecation; if the angle becomes more obtuse, it proves failure to completely widen during defecation
    • The degree of pelvic floor descent
    • Anatomic abnormalities, such as rectocele, solitary rectal ulcers, anal mucosal prolapse, or intussusception (17)
❖ Balloon expulsion test
  ◆ The balloon expulsion test is performed by inserting a latex balloon into the patient's rectum and then filling it up with 50 mL of water or air.
  ◆ It helps to quantify the ability of a patient to expel the balloon. Failure to do so within 2 minutes suggests a defecation dysfunction.
  ◆ It is usually combined with anorectal manometry that is described next.

Table 4. Anorectal Manometry

Measurement	Abnormality	Diagnostic Possibility
Resting external anal sphincter pressure	Increased	Anal fissure
Resting internal anal sphincter pressure	Increased	Obstructed constipation
Anorectal inhibitory reflex	Absent	Hirschsprung's disease
		Rectal enlargement from retained stool
Rectal sensation	Decreased	Neurologic disorder
		Prolonged retention of stool

❖ Anorectal manometry
  ◆ Anorectal manometry provides several useful measurements, as described in Table 4 (18).

Treatment

The first step in treatment of constipation is an increase in fluid intake and physical activity. This should be followed by increasing fiber intake to 20–25 g/day for a few weeks, either by incorporating more fiber into the diet or with commercial fiber supplements. Patients who do not respond to fiber therapy should begin treatment with a saline osmotic laxative, such as milk of magnesia. More expensive agents, such as lactulose and polyethylene glycol, should be reserved for patients who are refractory to fiber or osmotic laxatives.

Laxatives

❖ Laxatives can be grouped into two major categories—oral and rectal.
❖ The classification of oral laxatives according to their mode of action is illustrated in Figure 2 and Table 5.

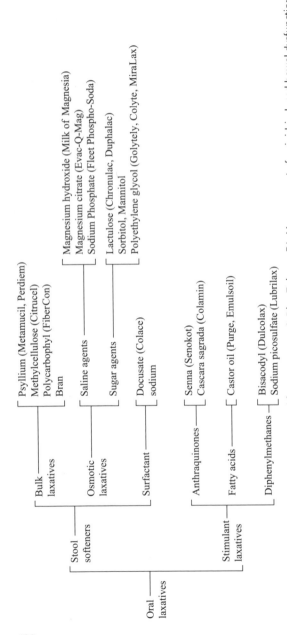

Figure 2. Classification of laxatives. (Adapted from Tamayo AC, Diaz-Zuluaga PA. Management of opioid-induced bowel dysfunction in cancer patients. Support Care Cancer 2004;12:613–618.)

Table 5. Medications Used for Constipation

Medication	Trade Name	Dose	Onset of Action	Mechanism of Action	Side Effects
Stool softeners					
Bulk laxatives				Increases stool bulk; decreases colonic transit time	
Psyllium	Metamucil® (Procter & Gamble), Perdiem® (Novartis Consumer)	1 tsp up to TID	12–72 h		Bloating, flatulence, fluid overload
Methylcellulose	Citrucel® (Mission)	1 tsp up to TID	12–72 h		Less bloating, flatulence, fluid overload
Polycarbophil	FiberCon® (Wyeth), Equalactin® (Corad)	2–4 tab qd	24–48 h		Bloating, flatulence, fluid overload
Bran		1 c qd			Bloating, flatulence, iron and calcium malabsorption

(continued)

Table 5. *Continued*

Medication	Trade Name	Dose	Onset of Action	Mechanism of Action	Side Effects
Osmotic laxatives				Fluid osmotically drawn into the intestines, decreases colonic transit time	
Saline laxatives					
Magnesium hydroxide	Phillips' Milk of Magnesia Bayer®	15–30 mL qd or BID	1–3 h		Hypermagnesemia, dehydration, abdominal cramps
Magnesium citrate		150–300 mL prn	0.5–3.0 h		Hypermagnesemia, dehydration, abdominal cramps
Sodium phosphate	Fleet Phospho-Soda® (Fleet)	10–25 mL			Hyperphosphatemia
Sugar laxatives				Nonabsorbable synthetic disaccharide metabolized by colonic bacteria into short-chain fatty acids; retains water and electrolytes by osmotic effect	
Lactulose	Duphalac® (Solvay)	15–30 mL qd or BID	24–48 h		Bloating, flatulence

Sorbitol		15–30 mL qd or BID	24–48 h		Bloating, flatulence
Mannitol		15–30 mL qd or BID	24–48 h		Bloating, flatulence
Polyethylene glycol (PEG)	Golytely® (Braintree), MiraLax® (Braintree)	17–36 g qd or BID	0.5–1.0 h	Poorly absorbed organic polymers not metabolized by colonic bacteria; retains water and electrolytes by osmotic effect	Less bloating and flatulence
Surfactant					
Docusate sodium	Colace® (Shire US)	100 mg BID	12–72 h	Lowers surface tension of stool, allowing water to enter stool	Skin rash
Stimulant laxatives					
Anthraquinones		Titrate for relief of symptoms		Increases intraluminal fluids; increases motility by stimulating myenteric plexus	Malabsorption, melanosis coli
Cascara sagrada		1–2 tab qd	6–12 h		
Senna	Senokot® (Senokot)	2–4 tab qd	6–12 h		

(continued)

Table 5. *Continued.*

Medication	Trade Name	Dose	Onset of Action	Mechanism of Action	Side Effects
Fatty acids					
Castor oil	Purge® (Fleming), Emulsoil® (Paddock)	15–30 mL qd		Hydrolyzed to ricinoleic acid; inhibits water absorption in the small intestine and stimulates motor function	Cramping, severe diarrhea
Diphenyl-methanes					
Bisacodyl	Dulcolax® (Boehringer)	10–30 mg PO qd 10-mg suppository qhs	6–10 h 15–60 min	Stimulates secretion and increases motility of small intestine and colon	Hyperkalemia, abdominal cramps
Sodium picosulfate	Lubrilax® (Normon)	5–15 mg qhs		Stimulates secretion and increases motility only of colon	
Lubricant					
Mineral oil	Fleet® Mineral Oil (Fleet)	5–15 ml qhs	6–8 h	Lubricates stool	Dehydration, malabsorption of fat-soluble vitamins, lipid pneumonia

Enemas				Initiates evacuation by softening hard stools and distending the rectum; topically stimulates contraction of colonic muscle	
Mineral oil retention enema	Fleet® mineral oil enema (Fleet)	100 mL qd	6–8 h		Incontinence, mechanical trauma
Phosphate enema	Fleet® enema (Fleet)	120 mL qd	5–15 min		Hyperphosphatemia, mechanical trauma
Tap water enema		500 mL qd	5–15 min		Mechanical trauma
Soapsuds enema		1,500 mL qd	2–15 min		Mechanical trauma
Prokinetic agent					
Tegaserod	Zelnorm® (Novartis)	6 mg BID		Induces peristalsis by stimulating 5-hydroxytryptamine receptors in the intestines (partial agonist)	
Miscellaneous					
Colchicine	Colsalide® (Vortech)	0.6 mg TID		Accelerates colonic transit	Diarrhea, neuromuscular complications
Misoprostol	Cytotec® (Searle)	600–2,400 mcg qd		Accelerates colonic transit	Diarrhea

Adapted from Locke GR 3rd, Pemberton JH, Phillips SF. AGA technical review on constipation. American Gastroenterological Association. Gastroenterology 2000;119:1766–1778.

135

❖ Rectal laxatives include suppositories, clysmas, and enemas that act by inhibiting the reabsorption of fluid and sodium from the bowel lumen or as stool softeners (Table 5).

Medications

❖ Prokinetic agents, such as tegaserod, improve stool consistency and frequency in patients with constipation as the predominant feature of IBS (19).

❖ Prostaglandin analogues, such as misoprostol, cause diarrhea as a major side effect and, hence, could be used to treat constipation. However, its cost-effectiveness limits its use (20).

❖ Colchicine increases the frequency of bowel movements and accelerates colonic transit. Hence, it can be used in patients with constipation refractory to other medications (21).

❖ Opioid antagonists, such as methylnaltrexone, reverse opioid-induced constipation by acting on the peripheral opioid receptors. It does not cross the blood–brain barrier and, hence, does not interfere with analgesia.

Biofeedback Therapy

❖ *Biofeedback therapy* encompasses visual and auditory feedback on functioning of a patient's anal sphincter and pelvic floor muscles.

❖ Patients' can be trained to relax the pelvic floor muscles along with appropriate coordination of the abdominal muscles during an act of defecation. The training can also be achieved with the aid of a silicon-filled artificial stool (22).

❖ Patient and therapist motivation, along with the development of a rapport, is the key to successful therapy.

Surgery

❖ Surgery should only be considered in patients with severe constipation when all medical therapies have failed.

❖ Total colectomy with ileorectal anastomosis is the preferred treatment for patients with slow transit constipation (3).

❖ Rectal surgery should be considered in patients with rectocele-induced constipation (23).

Diarrhea

Chemotherapeutic agents have been used in the fight against cancer for several years. These therapeutic agents have several side effects associated with them. Diarrhea is a severe side effect that can have increased risk of mortality compared with other regimens (24). In addition, as higher doses of chemotherapy are used, there can be a limitation on the oncologist to give the most optimal dose to the patient. The definition of diarrhea is dependent on three criteria: frequency greater than three bowel movements a day, consistency of the stool, and increased fecal weight (25).

Diarrhea is not limited to chemotherapeutics but is also present in adjunct therapies that an oncology patient may undergo. Radiation therapy is currently in use for several different cancers, and damage to the mucosa leads to profuse amounts of diarrhea. In addition, bone marrow patients not only undergo high doses of chemotherapy but are also prone to infections and graft-versus-host disease. The fragile condition of these patients can cause even minor episodes of diarrhea to be deadly.

Pathology

Several chemotherapeutic agents can lead to severe mucosal damage to the intestinal mucosa. Histopathologic studies of the intestinal mucosa have demonstrated several abnormalities related to chemotherapeutics. Specifically, 5-fluorouracil (5-FU) and CPT-11 were evaluated and demonstrated (26,27):

1. Acute damage to the mucosa
2. Prostaglandins, leukotrienes, cytokines, and free radicals stimulated secretions
3. Loss of brush border enzymes
4. Mitotic arrest and initiation of apoptosis in the crypts of the small intestine

These pathologic findings are for chemotherapeutic agents but with several other causes that can lead to slowing of peristalsis or infectious damage to the intestines. The etiology should be established before further workup is initiated.

Etiology

Diarrhea can occur in several different situations in the oncology patient. Some of these situations are as follows:

❖ Chemotherapeutic agents (Table 6)
❖ Decreased physical performance (activity decreased, decreased appetite, immobilization)
❖ Disease associated with therapy (i.e., graft-versus-host disease)

Table 6.   Chemotherapy-Induced Diarrhea

Chemotherapy	Incidence (Grade 3–4; %)
Capecitabine	30
Infusional 5-FU vs. bolus	12–21
Irinotecan/oxaliplatin	20
Oxaliplatin + infusional 5-FU/leucovorin	11
5-FU	
IV bolus	9
Continuous infusion	5
5-FU bolus +	
Low-dose leucovorin ($20\ mg/m^2$)	10
High-dose leucovorin ($200\ mg/m^2$)	23
CPT-11	
$100–125\ mg/m^2$	5–30
$150\ mg/m^2$	24
Topotecan	13

5-FU, 5-fluorouracil.
Adapted from Wadler S, Haynes H, Wiernik PH. Phase I trial of the somatostatin analog octreotide acetate in the treatment of fluoropyrimidine-induced diarrhea. J Clin Oncol 1995;13:222–226; and Farrell CL, Bready JV, Rex KL, et al. Keratinocyte growth factor protects mice from chemotherapy and radiation-induced gastrointestinal injury and mortality. Cancer Res 1998;58:933–939.

❖ Radiation therapy
❖ Infection (*Clostridium difficile*, parasites, viral)
❖ In addition, there are several factors that can lead to an increase in diarrhea that is already present:
   ◆ Inflammation due to other agents
   ◆ Infection
   ◆ Antibiotics

   Careful analysis of the causative agent can lead to more accurate management, and early intervention can help in preventing severe complications, which maybe irreversible.

Evaluation

The initial evaluation of the patient is extremely crucial. It is during the history and physical that a health care provider is able to assess the severity of the situation, so that the appropriate therapy can be started. During the history evaluation, questions about the duration, frequency, and quantity can provide valuable information to judge the severity of the problem (Table 7). The physical examination can add to the source of the diarrhea. It is important to evaluate antibiotics that the patient has taken in the past and the volume status of the patient. The laboratory evaluation can help to confirm the volume status of the patient, as well as whether electrolytes need to be repleted. In addition, a consultation may help to confirm or exclude a diagnosis of graft-versus-host disease in transplant patients. Also, infectious etiology (viral, bacterial, or fungal) has to be excluded, and the appropriate tests should be sent for culture.

   In addition, part of the history should include the medications that the patient is currently taking. Many herbal remedies and over-the-counter medications may cause diarrhea and should be inquired about. Dietary regimens can also lead to diarrhea when there are interactions with medication. Specifically, chemotherapeutic medication can lead to destruction of the gastric mucosa. Therefore, patients may not be able to absorb foods that were previously not leading to diarrhea. A thorough dietary history should

Table 7. Evaluation of Diarrhea

History	Physical Examination
Bowel-focused history	Hydration status
Onset	Vein filling
Duration	Blood urea nitrogen/creatinine
Frequency	Orthostatic hypotension
Aggravating or relieving factors	Mucosa
Stool-focused history	Abdominal examination
Volume	Soft/firm
Appearance	Tenderness
Consistency	Bowel sounds
Blood/mucus	Check ostomy if present
Odor	Rectal
Symptoms of dehydration	Hemorrhoids
Light-headedness	Periostomal
Thirst	Fissures
Decreased appetite	Infection
Fatigue	*Clostridium difficile*
General	Ova and parasites
Changes in weight	Stool culture
Comorbid conditions	Viruses in transplant patients
Medication	
Herbs, complementary therapies	

Adapted from Wadler S, Haynes H, Wiernik PH. Phase I trial of the somatostatin analog octreotide acetate in the treatment of fluoropyrimidine-induced diarrhea. J Clin Oncol 1995;13:222–226; Farrell CL, Bready JV, Rex KL, et al. Keratinocyte growth factor protects mice from chemotherapy and radiation-induced gastrointestinal injury and mortality. Cancer Res 1998;58:933–939; and Cao S, Troutt AB, Rustum YM. Interleukin 15 protects against toxicity and potentiates antitumor activity of 5-fluorouracil alone and in combination with leucovorin in rats bearing colorectal cancer. Cancer Res 1998;58:1695–1699.

be taken, and, if necessary, a dietitian should be consulted for recommendations.

Several oncology patients are neutropenic and need urgent treatment of severe diarrhea because it can be fatal. In addition,

Table 8. National Cancer Institute Common Terminology Criteria for Adverse Events

Grade	Interference with ADL	Without Colostomy	With Colostomy
1	No	Increase of <4 stools/day	Mild increase in output
2	No	Increase of 4–6 stools/day	Moderate increase in output
3	Yes	Increase of ≥7 stools/day	Severe increase in output
4	Yes	Hemodynamic collapse	
5		Death	

ADL, activities of daily living.
Adapted from de Roy van Zuidewijn DB, Schillings PH, Wobbes T, et al. Morphometric analysis of the effects of antineoplastic drugs on mucosa of normal ileum and ileal anastomoses in rats. Exp Mol Pathol 1992;56:96–107.

patients with colostomy bags are also at risk for diarrhea and should be monitored closely. The severity of diarrhea can be graded by the National Cancer Institute Common Toxicity Criteria (Table 8) (28). This allows for a common nomenclature, so that health care practitioners are able to have a unified method of describing diarrhea.

Initial evaluation can help to divide diarrhea into several different types, which can help to narrow the differential. The types of diarrhea are fatty, motility disorders, watery, and inflammatory (Table 9) (29). A preliminary analysis of the stool can be made by evaluating for the following:

1. Occult blood for tumors or infectious etiology, but this can be of questionable importance and should be followed up with further testing
2. White blood cells on initial Gram stain using Wright's stain
3. Sudan stain for fat
4. pH, electrolytes, and minerals
5. Fecal culture should be sent during the initial workup for patients

Table 9. Types of Diarrhea with Evaluation

Fatty	Motility	Inflammatory	Watery	
			Secretory	Osmotic
Greasy, floating, malodorous	Postsurgical disorders, masses, iatrogenic neuropathy	Blood and mucus		Usually medication induced, carbohydrate, magnesium
1. 72 h fecal fat	1. Subsides after fast, osmolality = 250–300	1. Infection	1. Continues despite fasting	
		a. *Clostridium difficile*	2. Day and night, no control	
		b. Parasites		
		c. Tuberculosis	1. Difference can be established by stool electrolytes	
		2. Fecal leukocytes	2. Stool cultures	
		3. Fecal calprotectin	3. Imaging of large and small bowel	
			4. Gastrin and VIP testing	
			5. Bile acid malabsorption	

VIP, vasoactive intestinal peptide.

Other workups of importance in the blood and urine are as follows:

❖ Urine

  1. Vanillylmandelic acid
  2. 5-Hydroxyindoleacetic acid
  3. Laxative

❖ Blood

  1. Vasoactive intestinal peptide
  2. Electrolytes
  3. Other peptides
  4. Vitamin B_{12}
  5. Pancreatic enzymes

Management of diarrhea is dictated by the severity of toxicity and the type of diarrhea.

Management

In some chemotherapeutic regimens, there is life-threatening diarrhea, and there are several ways that such diarrhea can be treated (Figure 3). The appropriate treatment of this diarrhea not only allows for better outcomes because patients are able to tolerate the regimen better, but it also helps improve the quality of life of the individuals. Nutritional therapy may also benefit some patients who present with acute diarrhea (Table 10).

After initial evaluation, patients may need fluid restoration and/ or admission to the hospital. Health care practitioners should keep in mind that the goal is not only to stop the diarrhea but to discover whether there is an underlying etiology that can be treated. In particular, infectious etiology may need to be treated before stopping the diarrhea. Also, the practitioner should pay special attention to determine whether an obstruction is the reason for the diarrhea. Caution should be used when dealing with refractory diarrhea, as a complete workup consisting of a gastroenterology consult may be necessary to determine whether cancer is the cause of the diarrhea (i.e., colon cancer or a carcinoid syndrome). If these factors have

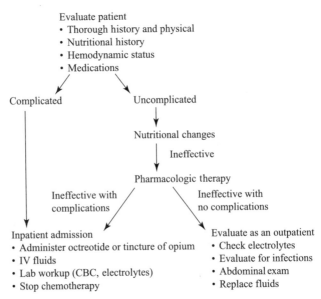

Figure 3
Management of chemotherapy-induced diarrhea. CBC, complete blood cell count.

Table 10.   Nutritional Guidelines for Acute Diarrhea

Benefit	Avoid
8–10 Large glasses of clear liquids	Spicy food
Eat small meals	Alcohol
Eat and drink plenty of foods to replace electrolytes and minerals	Dairy products
	High-osmolar products
Adequate soluble fiber	High-sugar drinks
Protein-rich foods	High-fat foods
Eat slowly	

Adapted from Lamberts SW, van der Lely AJ, de Herder WW, et al. Octreotide. N Engl J Med 1996;334:246–254; and Mercandante S. Diarrhea, malabsorption and constipation. In: Berger A, Portenoy RK, Weissman DE, eds. Principles and practice of supportive oncology, 2nd ed. Philadelphia: Lippincott Williams & Wilkins, 2002.

Table 11. Recommendations for Management of Chemotherapy-Induced Diarrhea: Pharmacologic Management after Nonpharmacologic Interventions Have Been Unsuccessful

Diarrhea, any NCI toxicity grade	Oral loperamide (see dosing)
Refractory to loperamide for more than 24 h	Oral fluoroquinolone for 7 days
Refractory to loperamide for more than 48 h	Admit patient to the hospital
	Stop loperamide
	Aggressive hydration
ANC <500 cells/mcL	Oral fluoroquinolone until not neutropenic
Fever with diarrhea	Oral fluoroquinolone continue until symptoms resolve
Refractory diarrhea	Octreotide, tincture of opium, discontinue chemotherapy

ANC, absolute neutrophil count; NCI, National Cancer Institute.
Adapted from Lamberts SW, van der Lely AJ, de Herder WW, et al. Octreotide. N Engl J Med 1996;334:246–254.

been excluded and it is appropriate after a thorough examination, then pharmacologic therapy (Table 11) can be started to limit the frequency and quantity of the diarrhea. As mentioned in the classification of antidiarrhea medications (Table 12), there are several mechanisms that can be used for the treatment of diarrhea.

It should be noted that opioids are extremely helpful medications in mild to moderate diarrhea management but are many

Table 12. Medications for Diarrhea

Antibiotics	Bile Acid Agents	Absorbents	Opiates	Other
Metronidazole	Bismuth	Clays	Tincture of opium	Anticholinergic medication
Amoxicillin	Medicinal fiber	Activated charcoal	Morphine	Octreotide
Neomycin/bacitracin	Cholestyramine	Psyllium	Codeine	Loperamide
				Budesonide

times overlooked. Specifically, tincture of opium and morphine may be more useful than codeine. In patients who may have excess bile acid secretions, bismuth, medicinal fiber, and cholestyramine may be of use. There are also several ways that the stool consistency may be changed by providing absorbents, such as clays, activated charcoal, or psyllium. The other option is that of steroids, such as budesonide, which has a low systemic absorption because of the first pass mechanism in the liver and is used in Crohn's disease (29). It should be kept in mind that using medications that are anticholinergics can be used as a last resort, but toxicity at higher doses should be taken into consideration.

Two popular medications for the treatment of chemotherapy-induced diarrhea are loperamide and octreotide.

Several experimental trials are currently ongoing with several different substances. Many of these experimental medications have explored preventive therapy for, as well as therapy to treat, specific chemotherapy-induced diarrheas. For example, oral glutamine, thalidomide, and oral neomycin/bacitracin are currently being investigated in irinotecan-induced diarrhea. There are also several substances that show promising results in animal studies. Keratinocyte growth factor has helped in proliferation and differentiation of epithelial cells. This has shown to be useful in animal models in the prevention of diarrhea (34). Also, interleukin-15 has shown promise in reducing chemotherapy-induced diarrhea in animal models (35).

Loperamide

Mechanism

- ❖ Antidiarrheal
- ❖ Inhibits peristalsis and prolongs transit time by acting on intestinal mucosa
- ❖ Enhances fluid and electrolyte movement through intestinal mucosa

Indication

- ❖ Mild to moderate uncomplicated diarrhea
- ❖ If not effective after 48 hours, then consider therapy with second-line medication

Dosing

- ❖ Initially, give 4 mg orally, then give 2 mg after each stool that is not formed. If the diarrhea persists past 24 hours, then an increase in dose is appropriate.
- ❖ If refractory to the initial dose, begin 2 mg every 2 hours until the patient is free of diarrhea for 12 hours (24).

Side Effects

- ❖ Increased risk of paralytic ileus; should monitor the patient closely
- ❖ Distension, cramping, bloating
- ❖ Dizziness, drowsiness, fatigue

Evidence

- ❖ Increased mortality in patients who were treated with irinotecan, 5-FU, and leucovorin because of increased risk of infection (24)

Octreotide

Mechanism

- ❖ Synthetic somatostatin analogue
- ❖ Acts on somatostatin receptors
- ❖ Used in several endocrine disorders (30)

Indication

- ❖ Moderate to severe diarrhea when more aggressive approach needed

Dosing

- ❖ Initially, 100–150 mcg subcutaneously three times a day, or intravenously (25–50 mcg/hour).
- ❖ If symptoms worsen, increase to 500 mcg until the diarrhea is controlled (31).
- ❖ Data support using up to 2,500 mcg three times daily.

Side Effects

- ❖ Bloating, flatulence, and cramping.
- ❖ Glucose should be monitored at higher doses because hyperglycemia may occur.

❖ Patients with cardiac history should be monitored for brady-cardia.

❖ Drug interactions should be monitored closely in the oncology population, and cyclosporine levels should be checked frequently because there may be a reduction in dose.

Evidence

❖ In addition, further studies have compared the 100-mcg dose to the 500-mcg dose and found increased efficacy in eliminating diarrhea without a greater number of side effects (32).

❖ In a trial of patients who received 5-FU or a modified 5-FU regimen, dose escalation up to 2,500 mcg three times a day was beneficial in stopping diarrhea (33).

References

1. Oi-Ling K, Man-Wah DT, Kam-Hung DN. Symptoms as rated by advanced care patients, care givers and physicians in the last week of life. Pall Med 2005;19:228–233.

2. Thompson WG, Creed F, Drossman DA, et al. Functional bowel disorders and functional abdominal pain. Gut 1999;45:1143–1147.

3. Nyam DC, Pemberton JH, Ilstrup DM, et al. Long-term results of surgery for chronic constipation. Dis Colon Rectum 1997;40:273–279.

4. Ashraf W, Park F, Lof J, et al. An examination of the reliability of reported stool frequency in the diagnosis of idiopathic constipation. Am J Gastroenterol 1996;91:26–32.

5. Voderholzer WA, Schatke W, Muhldorfer BE, et al. Clinical response to dietary fiber treatment of chronic constipation. Am J Gastroenterol 1997;92:95–98.

6. Preston DM, Lennard-Jones JE. Anismus in chronic constipation. Dig Dis Sci 1985;30:413–418.

7. Camilleri M, Thompson WG, Fleshman JW, et al. Clinical management of intractable constipation. Ann Intern Med 1994;121:520–528.

8. Preston DM, Lennard-Jones JE. Pelvic motility and response to intraluminal bisacodyl in slow-transit constipation. Dig Dis Sci 1985;30:289.

9. Bassotti G, Chiarioni G, Imbimbo BP, et al. Impaired colonic motor response to cholinergic stimulation in patients with severe chronic idiopathic (slow transit type) constipation. Dig Dis Sci 1993;38:1040–1045.

10. Tzavella K, Riepl RL, Klauser AG, et al. Decreased substance P levels in rectal biopsies from patients with slow transit constipation. Eur J Gastroenterol Hepatol 1996;8:1207–1211.

11. He CL, Burgart L, Wang L, et al. Decreased interstitial cell of Cajal volume in patients with slow transit constipation. Gastroenterology 2000;118:14–21.

12. Snape WJ Jr. Role of colonic motility in guiding therapy in patients with constipation. Dig Dis Sci 1997;15:104–111.

13. Mertz H, Naliboff B, Mayer E. Physiology of refractory chronic constipation. Am J Gastroenterol 1999;94:609–615.

14. Harewood GC, Coulie B, Camilleri M, et al. Descending perineum syndrome: audit of clinical and laboratory features and outcome of pelvic floor retaining. Am J Gastroenterol 1999;94:126–130.

15. Hinton JM, Lennard-Jones JE, Young AC. A new method for studying gut transit times using radioopaque markers. Gut 1969;10:842–847.

16. Wald A, Caruana BJ, Freimanis MG, et al. Contributions of evacuation proctography and anorectal manometry to the evaluation of adults with constipation and defecatory difficulty. Dig Dis Sci 1990; 35:481.

17. Schweiger M, Alexander-Williams J. Solitary rectal ulcer syndrome of the rectum: its association with occult rectal prolapse. Lancet 1977;1:1970–1971.

18. Diamant NE, Kamm MA, Wald A, et al. AGA technical review on anorectal testing techniques. Gastroenterology 1999;116:735–760.

19. Muller-Lissner SA, Fumagalli I, Bardhan KD, et al. Tegaserod, a 5-HT (4) receptor partial agonist, relieves symptoms in irritable bowel syndrome patients with abdominal pain, bloating and constipation. Aliment Pharmacol Ther 2001;15:1655–1666.

20. Soffer EE, Metcalf A, Launspach J. Misoprostol is effective treatment for patients with severe constipation. Dig Dis Sci 1994;39:929–933.

21. Verne GN, Davis RH, Robinson ME, et al. Treatment of chronic constipation with colchicine: randomized, double-blind, placebo-controlled, crossover trial. Am J Gastroeneterol 2003;98:1112–1116.

22. Pelsang RE, Rao SS, Welcher K. FECOM: a new artificial stool for evaluating defecation. Am J Gastroenterol 1999;94:183–186.

23. Sarles JC, Arnaud A, Selezneff I, et al. Endo-rectal repair of rectocele. Int J Colorectal Dis 1989;4:167–171.

24. Rothenberg ML, Meropol NJ, Poplin EA, et al. Mortality associated with irinotecan plus bolus fluorouracil/leucovorin: summary findings of an independent panel. J Clin Oncol 2001;19:3801–3807.

25. Wenzl HH, Fine KD, Schiller LR, et al. Determinants of decreased fecal consistency in patients with diarrhea. Gastroenterol 1995;108: 1729–1738.

26. Dosik GM, Luna M, Valdivieso M, et al. Necrotizing colitis in patients with cancer. Am J Med 1979;67:646–656.

27. de Roy van Zuidewijn DB, Schillings PH, Wobbes T, et al. Morphometric analysis of the effects of antineoplastic drugs on mucosa of normal ileum and ileal anastomoses in rats. Exp Mol Pathol 1992;56:96–107.

28. Cancer Therapy Evaluation Program, common terminology criteria for adverse events Version 3.0. 2003, NIH publication No. 03-5410.

29. Mercandante S. Diarrhea, malabsorption and constipation. In: Berger A, Portenoy RK, Weissman DE, eds. Principles and practice of supportive oncology, 2nd ed. Philadelphia: Lippincott Williams & Wilkins, 2002.

30. Lamberts SW, van der Lely AJ, de Herder WW, et al. Octreotide. N Engl J Med 1996;334:246–254.

31. Benson AB 3rd, Ajani JA, Catalano RB, et al. Recommended guidelines for the treatment of cancer treatment-induced diarrhea. J Clin Oncol 2004;22:2918–2926.

32. Goumas P, Naxakis S, Christopoulou A, et al. Octreotide acetate in the treatment of fluorouracil-induced diarrhea. Oncologist 1998;3:50-53.

33. Wadler S, Haynes H, Wiernik PH. Phase I trial of the somatostatin analog octreotide acetate in the treatment of fluoropyrimidine-induced diarrhea. J Clin Oncol 1995;13:222–226.

34. Farrell CL, Bready JV, Rex KL, et al. Keratinocyte growth factor protects mice from chemotherapy and radiation-induced gastrointestinal injury and mortality. Cancer Res 1998;58:933–939.

35. Cao S, Troutt AB, Rustum YM. Interleukin 15 protects against toxicity and potentiates antitumor activity of 5-fluorouracil alone and in combination with leucovorin in rats bearing colorectal cancer. Cancer Res 1998;58:1695–1699.

Oral Mucositis

Douglas E. Peterson, DMD, PhD

Scope of the Problem

Oral mucositis is a common toxicity of selected cytoreductive cancer therapies (1–4). Its clinical expression can range from mild discomfort without overt lesions to extensive, severely painful oral ulcerations (Figure 1). As discussed in more detail later, exposure of oral mucosa to high-dose radiation and/or chemotherapy results in a cascade of cellular and tissue events that collectively result in this mucosal injury. Incidence rates of clinically significant oral mucositis are summarized in Table 1 (5).

Severity of oral mucositis in head and neck cancer patients is directly governed by the radiation doses delivered to the tissues. Unlike chemotherapy-induced toxicity, oral mucositis caused by radiation occurs in the field of tissue that is irradiated. Current head and neck radiation regimens, with or without concurrent chemotherapy, virtually always produce at least World Health Organization grade 3 oral mucositis when oral mucosal fields are involved.

Chemotherapy-induced oral mucositis has more variable expression across patients and across oral mucosal anatomic sites. While it is uncommon for the hard palate and gingiva to be clinically involved, there are several frequently involved sites including the following locations:

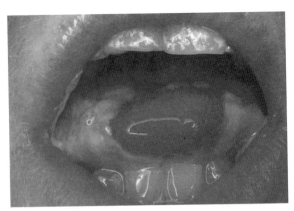

Figure 1
Oral mucositis in a high-dose chemotherapy patient. (Reprinted with permission from Dental Clinics of North America, V49(4), Lalla RV, et al: "Oral Mucositis" © 2005 Elsevier, Inc.)

- ❖ Buccal mucosa
- ❖ Floor of mouth
- ❖ Lateral tongue
- ❖ Soft palate

Reasons for this diversity are not well defined; the following are possible contributors:

- ❖ Tissue-based factors
  - ◆ Degree of keratinization
  - ◆ Tissue permeability
  - ◆ Epithelial cell replication rates
- ❖ Patient-based factors
  - ◆ Degree of oral health
  - ◆ Age of patient
  - ◆ History of previous chemotherapy treatment (6)

In chemotherapy patients, the most severe cases of oral mucositis tend to occur when certain classes and doses of agents are used [e.g., 5-fluorouracil (5-FU), methotrexate, and etoposide] (4) (Figure 2). Anthracycline-based regimens typically cause grade 3 oral mucositis in 1%–10% of patients, except when combined with 5-FU. Grade 3 oral mucositis caused by taxane- and platinum-based regimens typically occurs in <10% of patients, except when com-

Table 1.   Incidence of Oral Mucositis

Setting	Incidence (%)	Grades 3–4 (%)
Head and neck radiation	85–100	25–45
Stem cell transplant	75–100	25–60
Solid tumor, myelosuppressed patients	5–40	5–15

Adapted from Trotti A, Bellm LA, Epstein JB, et al. Mucositis incidence, severity and associated outcomes in patients with head and neck cancer receiving radiotherapy with or without chemotherapy: a systematic literature review. Radiother Oncol 2003;66:253–262; and Sonis ST, Elting LS, Keefe D, et al. Perspectives on cancer therapy-induced mucosal injury. Pathogenesis, measurement, epidemiology, and consequences for patients. Cancer 2004;100(9 Suppl):1995–2025.

bined with 5-FU or radiation. Rates of severe oral mucositis can be high in patients with gastrointestinal malignancies (53%; 95% confidence interval, 40%–44%, in four studies); this group often receives therapy based on 5-FU, CPT-11, and radiation.

Patients undergoing hematopoietic stem cell transplant (HSCT) frequently develop at least grade 3 oral mucositis. In adults, conditioning

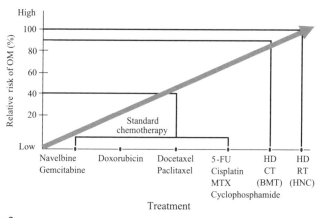

Figure 2
Relationship of oral mucositis (OM) incidence to ca   ncer therapy. Note: If patients develop OM during first chemotherapy cycle, risk of OM may increase in subsequent cycles. BMT, bone marrow transplant; CT, computed tomography; 5-FU, 5-fluorouracil; HD, high dose; HNC, head and neck cancer; MTX, methotrexate; RT, radiation therapy. (Courtesy of McNeil Pharmaceuticals.)

regimens can produce this degree of toxicity in approximately 25%–60% (5). The more severe lesions often occur in patients receiving melphalan. When total body irradiation is used as well, the rates increase to >60%. Although allogeneic transplant patients were historically reported to develop more severe oral mucositis than autologous patients did, current autologous conditioning regimens can also produce these more advanced toxicities. The impact of reduced-intensity conditioning regimens on oral mucositis in HSCT patients is less well defined in the literature, and requires additional investigation.

Oral mucositis contributes significantly to the quality of life of patients, including pain, nutritional compromise, and risk for systemic infection in neutropenic cancer patients. In a subset of patients, it can cause chemotherapy dose reduction or interruption of radiation therapy, resulting in risk for reduced patient survival (Figure 3). Complications of oral mucositis can also contribute to the cost of care. For example, Sonis et al. (7) have demonstrated that hospital charges averaged $42,749 more for HSCT patients with mucosal ulcerations compared with those without the lesions ($P = .06$). Costs included infection management, use of total parenteral nutrition, pain control with opioid narcotics, and extended hospital stays. Elting et al. (8) have conducted a health services study in 599 patients being treated with chemotherapy for solid tumors. Incremental costs associated with oral mucositis averaged approximately $2,384 per cycle, versus with no oral or gastrointestinal mucositis.

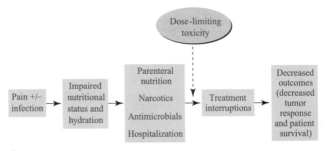

Figure 3
Potential impact of oral mucositis in cancer patients. (Courtesy of McNeil Pharmaceuticals.)

Contemporary Pathobiologic Model

Basic and translational research of oral mucositis has evolved over the past 15 years from identification of the need for study of mechanisms of injury to oral mucosa (9) to, more recently, novel research strategies for alimentary tract mucositis, including oral and gastrointestinal tissues (2). These advances have in turn lead to the paradigm of the impact of alimentary tract mucositis in relation to symptom clusters (10–12), as well as to development of clinical guidelines for management (13). This evolution has contributed to a conceptual shift in how investigators and clinicians envision the causation of mucosal injury in cancer patients, as well as in novel therapies directed toward molecular targets. As discussed in more detail later (see Treatment), the December 2004 U.S. Food and Drug Administration approval of keratinocyte growth factor-1 (palifermin) represents the first of potentially several new drugs to reduce the severity of oral and gastrointestinal mucositis.

For many decades, oral mucositis was viewed as primarily a direct result of injury to replicating oral basal epithelial cells by cytoreductive cancer therapy. Although this tissue remains a primary site for the toxicity, pathobiologic modeling that has evolved since the mid-1990s has produced new insights into the complexity of the lesion (14). The current model identifies molecular, cellular, and tissue changes in the epithelium, as well as underlying connective tissue that is altered throughout the continuum of injury and healing (4). Thus, oral mucositis can be viewed as a trans-tissue phenomenon. This biologic cross talk among diverse tissues and cell types is initiated within hours of the first administration of chemotherapy or radiation therapy and is characterized by a multifaceted inflammatory cascade governed by genetic expression (15). The current model is summarized in Table 2 (4).

Although the five phases interact in a temporally linear way, it is likely there is considerable interaction among the five phases throughout the period of inflammatory changes and tissue recovery. As noted earlier, this modeling has permitted pursuit of development of novel pharmacologic therapies for the toxicity. Given the pathobiologic complexity, it is therefore also likely that combination drug therapies will result in optimal reduction of severity in the future. This concept speaks to the critical importance of continued develop-

Table 2.   Current Pathobiologic Model of Oral Mucositis

Initiation

    Occurs within hours of initial exposure to cytotoxic cancer therapy

    Direct damage to epithelial DNA

    Generation of reactive oxygen species that promote a cascade of subsequent inflammatory events

    Clinical signs and symptoms not evident

Upregulation and message generation

    Occurs within the first several days of initial cancer therapy dosing.

    Activation of transcription factors (e.g., NF-κB) that in turn result in production of proinflammatory cytokines (e.g., TNF-α, IL-1β).

    These proinflammatory cytokines can cause direct tissue injury as well as apoptosis.

    Early mild pain symptoms and mild erythema may become evident late in this phase (e.g., 5–7 days after initiation of cancer therapy).

Amplification and signaling

    Occurs approximately 1 wk after initiation of cancer therapy; for chemotherapy patients, injury typically continues for several days after cessation of cancer therapy

    Generation of feedback loops that further escalate production of proinflammatory cytokines

Ulceration

    Typically occurs 7–10 days after initiation of cancer therapy.

    Classic and most severe expression of oral mucositis.

    Primary basis for clinical and economic impact, based on pain and infection risk.

    Metabolic products of bacterial cell walls can promote stimulation of macrophage-based inflammation biology.

Healing

    Occurs 2–4 wk after discontinuation of chemotherapy or radiation therapy

    Is governed by regulator proteins in the extracellular matrix and related processes

    Is characterized by migration, proliferation, and maturation of new mucosal epithelium

    Symptoms gradually resolve as the oral mucosal barrier becomes intact

IL-1β, interleukin-1β; TNF-α, tumor necrosis factor-α.

ment of drugs such that the clinician can customize therapies in the future based on risk of severity of oral mucositis. This approach is consistent with strategies used since the 1980s for the development of drugs to control nausea and emesis, which has resulted in often very effective therapies for reduction of these toxicities.

Labial mucosa, buccal mucosa, tongue, floor of mouth, and soft palate are more severely affected by chemotherapy than attached, heavily keratinized tissues, such as hard palate and gingiva; this may be due to their faster rate of epithelial cell turnover. Topical cryotherapy may ameliorate mucositis caused by agents, such as 5-FU, by reducing vascular delivery of these toxic agents to replicating oral epithelium. It is difficult to predict whether a patient will develop mucositis strictly on the basis of the classes of drugs that are administered. As suggested previously, several drugs are associated with propensity to damage oral mucosa; these include the following:

- ❖ Methotrexate
- ❖ Doxorubicin
- ❖ 5-FU
- ❖ Busulfan
- ❖ Bleomycin
- ❖ Platinum-based regimens complexes, including cisplatin and carboplatin

Patients who experience mucositis with a specific chemotherapy regimen during the first cycle appear to develop comparable mucositis during subsequent courses of that regimen.

Diagnosis

Use of accurate terminology is important to correctly diagnose oral mucositis in a clinical setting. Historically, mucositis and stomatitis have been often used synonymously. However, they are not homologous toxicities from a pathobiologic, as well as clinical, perspective. *Mucositis* refers to inflammatory conditions of the mucosa. *Stomatitis* refers to inflammatory conditions of the oral cavity. Thus, stomatitis may include mucositis, but it also includes other oral complications, including infection, salivary compromise, and chemosensory disturbances.

As described earlier (see Pathobiology), the initial symptoms and signs of oral mucositis begin approximately 5 days after initiation of cancer therapy. These typically include a mild burning sensation and mild erythema. Knowledge of treatment- and patient-based risk factors is important in counseling the patient and caregiver in advance, as well as in monitoring the patient's oral and systemic status in the early days after cancer treatment.

Several assessment scales are available for use by the clinician and investigator. These instruments vary in their complexity. Most patient care–based assessments use instruments that collectively assess symptoms, signs, and functional disturbances (National Cancer Institute Common Terminology Criteria for Adverse Events v. 3.0). Although these scales are often used to measure primary endpoints in clinical research settings for phase III investigations, other scales (e.g., Oral Mucositis Index, Oral Mucositis Assessment Scale) (16–18) may be used in phase II studies so that more detailed data regarding extent of tissue injury can be collected (4). Regardless of the type of assessment tool, it is important that the health professional using the instrument be trained in its use, as well as in the techniques to perform a systematic oral examination.

The diagnosis of oral mucositis thus incorporates knowledge of terminology and pathobiology combined with clinical assessment of symptoms and signs. Table 3 summarizes this model (19).

Treatment

The principles of supportive care management of oral mucositis include the following (20–24):

- ❖ Patient education and compliance
- ❖ Basic mouth care
- ❖ Nonmedicated saline rinses
- ❖ Topical and systemic pain control
- ❖ Hydration
- ❖ Nutritional support
- ❖ Infection surveillance and treatment

Table 3.   Diagnostic Approach for Oral Mucositis

Clinical appearance
  Initial erythematous appearance, followed by ulceration with or without pseudomembranous component

Symptoms
  Pain, with compromised oral functions in more severe cases

History of stomatotoxic therapy
  Clinical onset approximately 5 days after initiation of cancer therapy
    Previous cycles of cancer therapy may predispose the patient to more severe oral mucositis in subsequent cycles

Timing of onset of ulcerative component
  Ulcerations typically occur 7–10 days after initiation of cancer therapy

Duration of lesions
  Lesions usually resolve 2–4 wk after cessation of cancer therapy

Location of lesions
  Nonkeratinized oral mucosa is usually involved
    Chemotherapy patient
      Floor of mouth, lateral tongue, buccal and labial mucosa, soft palate
    Radiation patient
      Oral tissue receiving at least 3,000 centigrays, with nonkeratinized tissue more susceptible than keratinized sites.

Modified from Lalla RV and Peterson DE. Oral mucositis. Dent Clin N Am 2005;49:167–184.

There are a limited number of prospectively designed studies that document the role of basic, nonmedicated oral care in relation to mucositis risk and severity. However, systematic interventions several times per day (e.g., three times a day) are justified in the context of basic oral hygiene and wound care. These interventions are often based on bland rinses, as cited in Table 4.

Additional interventions can be introduced in a stepwise order, as symptoms and signs initially appear and then escalate. The frequency of baseline oral care can increase until wound care is being performed approximately six times per day. During this

Table 4. Supportive Care Interventions for Oral Mucositis

Soft toothbrush

Bland rinses

    0.9% Saline solution (swish and expectorate approximately 1 tbs several times per day)

    Sodium bicarbonate solution (swish and expectorate approximately 1 tbs several times per day, if viscous saliva is present)

    0.9% Saline/sodium bicarbonate solution

Topical anesthetics

    (Note: Having the patient perform an oral rinse with 0.9% saline solution immediately before administering these agents may enhance drug delivery, by removing loosely adherent oral debris and saliva)

    Lidocaine (viscous, ointments, sprays)

    Benzocaine (sprays, gels)

    0.5% or 1.0% dyclonine hydrochloride

    Diphenhydramine solution

Mucosal coating agents

    Amphojel® (Wyeth-Ayerst)

    Kaopectate® (Pfizer)

    Hydroxypropyl methylcellulose film-forming agents (e.g., Zilactin®, Zila)

    Cyanoacrylate mucoadherent film

    Gelclair (approved by the FDA as a device)

Analgesics

    Benzydamine HCl topical rinse (not approved in the United States)

    Opioid drugs [oral, intravenous (e.g., bolus, continuous infusion, patient-controlled analgesia)], patches, transmucosal

Growth factor (keratinocyte growth factor-1)

    Palifermin

        Approved by the FDA in December 2004 to decrease the incidence and duration of severe oral mucositis in patients undergoing high-dose chemotherapy with or without radiation therapy followed by bone marrow transplant for hematologic cancers

FDA, U.S. Food and Drug Administration.
Adapted from Oral complications of chemotherapy and head/neck radiation. National Cancer Institute. Available at: http://www.nci.nih.gov/cancertopics/pdq/ supportivecare/oralcomplications/healthprofessional. Accessed September 7, 2005.

time, the following continue to be hallmarks of patient management (Table 4):

❖ Pain control
❖ Nutritional support
❖ Infection surveillance and treatment

Evidence-based guidelines for the management of oral and/or gastrointestinal mucositis were published in 2004 by members of the Multinational Association for Supportive Care in Cancer and the International Association for Oral Oncology (13) (Table 5). Although these guidelines are not designed to completely replace the standard approaches that have been used (see Table 4), they do represent comprehensive, contemporary approaches that have been systematically evaluated based on the literature. These guidelines emerged from the evaluation of more than 8,000 publications from 1966 to 2001; the resulting recommendations were based on criteria published by the American Society of Clinical Oncology (25). In 2005, the mucositis guidelines were undergoing updating, with anticipated publication in 2006.

As noted previously in this paper, palifermin (keratinocyte growth factor-1) has been approved by the U.S. Food and Drug Administration to decrease the incidence and duration of severe oral mucositis in patients with hematologic cancers who are undergoing high-dose chemotherapy, with or without radiation therapy, followed by a bone marrow transplant. This first in-class approval represents a strategically important opportunity to reduce oral mucositis in this high-risk group of patients based on data in an autologous bone marrow transplant cohort (26) (Table 6). The concept of customizing mucositis management strategies continues to have potential. In this model, orally administered agents can be used for low- to moderate-risk patients. A combination of orally and systemically administered agents could be used for higher-risk patients. These strategies, however, need to be based on the following two parameters:

1. Additional drugs receive U.S. Food and Drug Administration approval in the coming years
2. Extensive phase IV testing, including safety

Table 5.   Clinical Practice Guidelines for Care of Patients with Oral Mucositis (Developed by the Multinational Association of Supportive Care in Cancer and the International Society for Oral Oncology)

Foundations of care

> The panel suggests the use of oral care protocols that include patient education in an attempt to reduce the severity of mucositis from chemotherapy or radiation therapy.

> The panel recommends patient-controlled analgesia with morphine as the treatment of choice for oral mucositis pain in patients undergoing HSCT.

Radiotherapy, *prevention*

> To reduce mucosal injury, the panel recommends the use of midline radiation blocks and three-dimensional radiation treatment.

> The panel recommends benzydamine for prevention of radiation-induced mucositis in patients with head and neck cancer receiving moderate-dose radiotherapy.

> > (Note: Benzydamine hydrochloride is not approved for use in the United States.)

> The panel recommends that chlorhexidine not be used to prevent oral mucositis in patients with solid tumors of the head and neck who are undergoing radiotherapy.

Standard-dose chemotherapy, *prevention*

> The panel recommends that patients receiving bolus 5-FU chemotherapy undergo 30-min oral cryotherapy to prevent oral mucositis.

> The panel suggests using 20–30-min oral cryotherapy in an attempt to decrease mucositis in patients treated with bolus doses of edatrexate.

> The panel recommends that acyclovir and its analogues not be used routinely to prevent mucositis.

Standard-dose chemotherapy, *treatment*

> The panel recommends that chlorhexidine not be used to treat established oral mucositis.

High-dose chemotherapy with or without TBI plus HSCT, *prevention*

> The panel does not recommend the use of pentoxifylline to prevent mucositis in patients undergoing HSCT.

Table 5. *Continued*

Low-level laser therapy (LLLT) requires expensive equipment and specialized training. Because of interoperator variability, clinical trials are difficult to conduct, and their results are difficult to compare; nevertheless, the panel is encouraged by the accumulating evidence in support of LLLT. For centers capable of supporting the necessary technology and training, the panel suggests the use of LLLT in an attempt to reduce the incidence of oral mucositis and its associated pain in patients receiving high-dose chemotherapy or chemoradiotherapy before HSCT.

5-FU, 5-fluorouracil; HSCT, hematopoietic stem cell transplant; TBI, total body irradiation.
Note: In December 2004, the U.S. Food and Drug Administration approved palifermin for patients with hematologic malignancies who are undergoing high-dose chemotherapy, with or without radiation, followed by bone marrow transplant. The guidelines are being revised to reflect this and related evidence-based updates.
From Rubenstein EB, Peterson DE, Schubert M, et al. Clinical practice guidelines for the prevention and treatment of cancer therapy-induced oral and gastrointestinal mucositis. Cancer 2004;100(9 Suppl):2030, with permission.

Evidence exists that capsaicin preparations may help moderate pain secondary to oral mucositis (27). Stimulation of polymodal nociceptors by the product can produce elevation in the pain threshold. This threshold can be additionally increased by gradually increasing the capsaicin concentration via repeated applications. However, this approach may not be feasible or tolerable for patients with more advanced cases of oral mucositis. Further research is needed.

Future Directions

The pathobiologic model for oral mucositis has provided a compelling foundation for drug development collectively directed to the multiple phases of oral mucositis. In addition, the impact of

Table 6.   Palifermin for Oral Mucositis after Intensive Therapy for Hematologic Cancers Followed by Bone Marrow Transplant

Study design
High-dose chemotherapy, TBI, autologous PBSC
60 mcg/kg/day, 3 days pre-TBI, 3 days post-PBSC
Phase III trial
Percent of patients with WHO grade 4 oral mucositis
Placebo (N = 106) 62%
Palifermin (N = 106) 20% (<0.001)
Palifermin
Reduced the severity of oral mucositis
Improved the quality of life
Reduced health resource use

PBSC, peripheral blood stem cell; TBI, total body irradiation; WHO, World Health Organization.
Data from Spielberger R, Stiff P, Bensinger W, et al. Palifermin for oral mucositis after intensive therapy for hematologic cancers. N Engl J Med 2004;351:2590–2598.

reduced oral mucosal toxicity on gastrointestinal and other consequences of cancer therapy represents a provocative and important new direction for laboratory and clinical research. Figure 4 summarizes selected current drugs in development for oral mucositis, based on multiphase model of the toxicity.

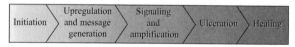

- Palifermin
- AES-14
- RK-0202
- CG53135
- Amifostine

Figure 4
Investigational drugs directed to the oral mucositis pathobiologic model.

❖ In addition to the U.S. Food and Drug Administration approval for bone marrow transplant patients as noted earlier, palifermin continues to undergo additional clinical trial testing in other cancer patients at significant risk for oral mucositis.

❖ AES-14 has completed one phase III study (28). The product represents technology designed to efficiently deliver high doses of L-glutamine, a conditionally essential amino acid, to oral mucosal tissue at risk for injury.

❖ RK-0202 is currently in phase II testing. The product is designed to scavenge reactive oxygen species generated by cancer therapy via N-acetylcysteine administered orally in a thermosetting gel.

❖ CG53135 is currently in phase II testing in transplant patients. This fibroblastic growth factor has bioactivity on epithelial and submucosal tissues.

❖ Amifostine is undergoing clinical testing for oral, esophageal, and intestinal mucositis. It is approved by the U.S. Food and Drug Administration for protection of salivary gland injury in head and neck cancer patients receiving radiation to the oral cavity.

Summary

There have been important advances in the pathobiologic modeling and multiprofessional approach to oral mucositis since the mid-1990s. The stage is now well set to continue drug development targeted toward the multiple etiologic components of the toxicity. Traditional interventions continue to be important in the overall management of the patient. U.S. Food and Drug Administration regulatory approval of new drugs in the coming years could position the oncology health professional to tailor the preventive and treatment approaches for the oral mucositis, based on risk for severity of the lesion.

References

1. Peterson DE. Research advances in oral mucositis. Curr Opin Oncol 1999;11:261–266.

2. Sonis ST, Peterson DE, McGuire DB, eds. Mucosal injury in cancer patients: new strategies for research and treatment. J Natl Cancer Inst Monogr 2001;(29):1–54.

3. McGuire DB, Peterson DE. Mucositis. Sem Oncol Nurs 2004;20:1–69.

4. Sonis ST, Elting LS, Keefe D, et al. Perspectives on cancer therapy-induced mucosal injury. Pathogenesis, measurement, epidemiology, and consequences for patients. Cancer 2004;100(9 Suppl):1995–2025.

5. Trotti A, Bellm LA, Epstein JB, et al. Mucositis incidence, severity and associated outcomes in patients with head and neck cancer receiving radiotherapy with or without chemotherapy: a systematic literature review. Radiother Oncol 2003;66:253–262.

6. Barasch A, Peterson DE. Risk factors for ulcerative oral mucositis in cancer patients: unanswered questions. Oral Oncol 2003;29:91–100.

7. Sonis ST, Oster G, Fuchs H, et al. Oral mucositis and the clinical and economic outcomes of hematopoietic stem-cell transplantation. J Clin Oncol 2001;19:2201–2205.

8. Elting LS, Cooksley C, Chambers M, et al. The burdens of cancer therapy. Clinical and economic outcomes of chemotherapy-induced mucositis. Cancer 2003;1:1531–1539.

9. Concensus Development Panel. Consensus Development Conference on oral complications of cancer therapies: Diagnosis, prevention, and treatment. J Natl Cancer Inst 1990;9:7.

10. Lee B-N, Dantzer R, Langley KE, et al. A cytokine-based neuroimmunologic mechanism of cancer-related symptoms. Neuroimmunomodulation 2004;11:279–292.

11. Keefe DM. Gastrointestinal mucositis: a new biological model. Supp Care Cancer 2004;12:6–9.

12. Elting LS, Keefe DMK, Sonis ST. Treatment-induced gastrointestinal toxicity in patients with cancer. Educational Session, 40th annual meeting, American Society of Clinical Oncology. 2004 Educational Book. 2004:536–541.

13. Rubenstein EB, Peterson DE, Schubert M, et al. Clinical practice guidelines for the prevention and treatment of cancer therapy-induced oral and gastrointestinal mucositis. Cancer 2004;100(9 Suppl):2026–2046.

14. Sonis ST. Mucositis as a biological process: a new hypothesis for the development of chemotherapy-induced stomatotoxicity. Oral Oncol 1998;34:39–43.

15. Sonis ST, Scherer J, Phelan S, et al. The gene expression sequence of radiated mucosa in an animal mucositis model. Cell Prolif 2002; 35(Suppl 1):93–102.

16. Schubert MM, Williams BE, Lloid ME, et al. Clinical assessment scale for the rating of oral mucosal changes associated with bone marrow transplantation. Development of an oral mucositis index. Cancer 1992; 69:2469–2477.

17. Sonis ST, Eilers JP, Epstein JB, et al. Validation of a new scoring system for the assessment of clinical trial research of oral mucositis induced by radiation or chemotherapy. Mucositis Study Group. Cancer 1999;85:2103–2113.

18. McGuire DB, Peterson DE, Muller S, et al. The 20 item oral mucositis index: reliability and validity in bone marrow and stem cell transplant patients. Cancer Invest 2002;20:893–903.

19. Lalla RV, Peterson DE. Oral mucositis. Dent Clin N Am 2005;49:167–184.

20. Larson PJ, Miaskowski C, MacPhail L, et al. The PRO-SELF Mouth Aware program: an effective approach for reducing chemotherapy-induced mucositis. Cancer Nurs 1998;21(4):263–268.

21. Kostler WJ, Hejna M, Wenzel C, et al. Oral mucositis complicating chemotherapy and/or radiotherapy: options for prevention and treatment. CA Cancer J Clin 2001;51:290–315.

22. Shih A, Miaskowski C, Dodd M, et al. A research review of the current treatments for radiation-induced oral mucositis in patients with head and neck cancer. Oncol Nurs Forum 2002;29:1063–1078.

23. Worthington HV, Clarkson JE, Eden OB. Interventions for treating oral mucositis for patients with cancer receiving treatment. Cochrane Database Syst Rev 2004;(2):CD001973.

24. Oral complications of chemotherapy and head/neck radiation. National Cancer Institute Web Site. Available at: http://www.nci.nih.gov/cancer-topics/pdq/supportivecare/oralcomplications/healthprofessional. Accessed September 7, 2005.

25. Somerfield M, Padberg J, Pfister D, et al. ASCO clinical practice guidelines: process, progress, pitfalls, and prospects. Classic Paper Curr Comments 2000;4:881–886.

26. Spielberger R, Stiff P, Bensinger W, et al. Palifermin for oral mucositis after intensive therapy for hematologic cancers. N Engl J Med 2004; 351:2590–2598.

27. Berger A, Henderson M, Nadoolman W, et al. Oral capsaicin provides temporary relief for oral mucositis pain secondary to chemotherapy/radiation therapy. J Pain Symptom Manage 1995;10:243–248.

28. Peterson DE, Petit RG. Phase III study: AES-14 in patients at risk for mucositis secondary to anthracycline-based chemotherapy. J Clin Oncol 2004;22(14S):abstract #8008.

Depression and Anxiety

Jimmie Holland, MD, and Soenke Boettger, MD

Depression and anxiety are common in the cancer care setting, and cancer patients are vulnerable to them at all stages of the illness. Cancer represents a major threat to the individual's well-being, and depressive and anxious responses are appropriate reactions. Although many cancer patients cope well with their illness, others experience a spectrum of depression and anxiety symptoms, which often interfere with function and ability to comply with cancer treatment. Psychiatric disorders occur in up to 50% of all cancer patients; most are represented by a mix of depression and anxiety symptoms, most of which are situationally related. This chapter outlines the major symptoms of each and the best treatment strategies.

❖ Depression and anxiety occur commonly in the cancer setting.

Depression

Cancer patients are at risk of developing depression at any stage of the illness:

❖ At appearance of the first symptoms of illness
❖ At diagnosis
❖ During treatment
❖ During palliative care

It even occurs in those surviving cancer. The prevalence of depression in cancer patients ranges from 25% to 42% (1).

Mood disorders (depressive symptoms) are among the most common forms of distress in cancer patients. *Depression* is best understood as a syndrome, which may range from a depressive reaction (called *adjustment disorder*) to the stress of illness to more severe symptoms of a major depressive disorder. Symptoms of cancer itself and some treatments produce depressive symptoms, which in the fourth edition of the *Diagnostic and Statistical Manual of Mental Disorders* (DSM-IV) is called *mood disorder due to general medical condition*. Some patients have a pre-existing chronic depression called *dysthymia*, which may become worse during illness (2).

Adjustment disorder with depressed mood (often with anxiety symptoms as well) represents difficulty in coping with an overwhelming situation. It often resolves with time and support. Major depressive disorder, however, often requires psychiatric intervention and should include evaluation of suicidal risk. Depressed mood due to cancer per se (e.g., paraneoplastic disorder) or drugs (e.g., steroids) requires management when the underlying process cannot be changed (3).

Signs, Symptoms, and Diagnosis of Depression

Depression is diagnosed by psychological and physical symptoms (see Table 1 for DSM-IV criteria for depressive diagnoses) (2). The primary psychological symptoms are as follows:

- ❖ Depressed or irritable mood
- ❖ Anhedonia (loss of pleasure)
- ❖ Feelings of hopelessness
- ❖ Worthlessness or guilt
- ❖ Low self-esteem
- ❖ Suicidal ideation

Physical signs of depression are similar to common symptoms caused by cancer and, hence, are less helpful than psychological symptoms in making the diagnosis. They include the following:

- ❖ A diminished ability to think or concentrate
- ❖ Lack of energy and fatigue
- ❖ Sleeping disturbance (usually insomnia)
- ❖ Anorexia

Table 1. DSM-IV Criteria for Common Depressive Disorders

Diagnosis	DSM-IV Criteria

Adjustment disorder
  With depressed mood
  With depressed/anxious mood
  Acute <6 mo
  Chronic >6 mo
	A. Development of emotional symptoms in response to an identifiable stressor (including illness) occurring within 3 mo
	B1. Marked distress that is greater than expected
	B2. Significant impairment in social or occupational functioning

Major depressive disorder Criterion 1 or 2, and at least four more criteria over at least 2 wk	1. Depressed mood *or* 2. Diminished interest or pleasure in activities and 3. Weight and appetite loss 4. Insomnia or hypersomnia 5. Psychomotor agitation or retardation 6. Fatigue or loss of energy 7. Feelings of worthlessness or guilt 8. Decreased concentration or indecisiveness 9. Recurrent thoughts of death
Mood disorder due to general medical condition—depressed prominent, persistent disturbance in mood	A. Depressed mood or markedly diminished interest and pleasure B. Mood disturbance is physiologically related to medical condition or medication

DSM-IV, *Diagnostic and Statistical Manual of Mental Disorders*, 4th edition.
Adapted from American Psychiatric Association. Diagnostic and Statistical Manual of Mental Disorders, 4th ed. Washington, DC: American Psychiatric Association, 1994.

❖ Weight loss
❖ Psychomotor slowing

The psychosocial predictors of poor coping with greater vulnerability to depressive symptoms are as follows:

❖ Social isolation
❖ Low socioeconomic status
❖ Alcohol or drug abuse
❖ Prior psychiatric history

- ❖ Prior experience with cancer (e.g., death of a relative)
- ❖ Recent losses/bereavement
- ❖ Inflexibility and rigidity of coping
- ❖ Pessimistic philosophy of life
- ❖ Absence of a belief/value system from which to view life and death
- ❖ Multiple obligations

Adjustment Disorder with Depressed Mood

Isolated depressive symptoms (which may be accompanied by anxiety symptoms) in response to stresses related to the illness result in a picture of reactive or situational depression called *adjustment disorder with depressed mood*. Mild to moderate symptoms may abate when the crisis is over, but more severe symptoms may persist and require medication, as well as support (4).

Major Depressive Disorder

Major depressive disorder is seen in up to 20%–25% of patients with cancer, depending on the stage of illness. It is far more common in patients with advanced disease and in hospitalized patients with significant disability. Treatment is usually indicated (3,5).

Mood Disorder Due to Cancer or Treatment

The DSM-IV classification calls depression due to a physiological cause (e.g., anemia) or a drug [e.g., steroids (6), interferon (7)] a mood disorder due to medical condition. The physical symptoms of fatigue, weakness, and depressed mood are most prominent. The effect of proinflammatory cytokines [interleukin-2 (IL-2), IL-6, IL-10] has been found to produce poor concentration, depressed and anxious mood, fatigue, and weakness. This has been termed *sickness behavior*, as noted in animals (8,9). This immunologic basis for common symptoms associated with depression is important to note.

Etiology

Causes of depression in cancer are related to psychosocial, physical, and physiologic factors. Table 2 outlines the common causes of depression in patients with cancer. The presence of uncontrolled

Table 2. Common Causes of Depression (Mood Disorders Due to General Medical Condition) in Cancer

Cancers and treatment	CNS metastases
	Primary brain tumor
	Paraneoplastic syndrome
	Pancreatic cancers
	Chemotherapeutics
	Asparaginase
	Mithramycin
	Vincristine
	Vinblastine
	Bleomycin
	Procarbazine
	Tamoxifen
Neurologic diseases	Cerebrovascular changes
	Cerebral trauma
	CNS infections
	Dementia
Metabolic abnormalities	Vitamin deficiencies
	Electrolyte imbalance
Endocrine disorders	Adrenal changes
	Thyroid function
Systemic disorders	Autoimmune disorders
	Inflammatory disorders
	Viral and other infections
Medications	Cardiac and antiarrhythmic drugs
	Steroids
	Antibiotics and antivirals
	Psychotropic drugs
	Neuroleptics
	Benzodiazepines
	Sedatives/hypnotics
	Neurologic agents
	Analgesics and anti-inflammatory drugs
	Opiates

(continued)

Table 2. *Continued*

Associated symptoms	Anemia
	Uncontrolled pain
	Cardiorespiratory disease
	Renal disease

CNS, central nervous system.

pain is a major cause of depression. Metabolic disorders and a range of medications contribute as well. A family history of depression or a history of personal depression predicts a greater vulnerability to having a depressive episode (10).

Management

Two treatment approaches are common in cancer. Nonpharmacologic interventions are those providing emotional support, counseling, psychotherapy, and complementary therapies, such as relaxation and meditation. They are helpful to many patients with depression (11). Pharmacologic interventions (Table 3) are required for the treatment of more severe adjustment disorders and major depression. A rapid onset of action is desirable in patients with cancer. Drug effects, interactions, and possible side effect profiles determine the choice of medication. A drug–drug interaction (e.g., inhibition of P450) is a consideration because it may interfere with metabolism of chemotherapeutic agents (12). Antidepressants are the mainstay of treatment in depressive disorders, and selective serotonin reuptake inhibitors (SSRIs) are most widely used. A major disadvantage of all antidepressants is the delayed onset of action, which may take as long as several weeks to have a therapeutic effect (13). For this reason, and the desire for a rapid onset to reduce symptoms, an antianxiety or neuroleptic drug may be given to produce an immediate effect while waiting for the slower onset of action of the antidepressant. Antidepressants should be started at low doses in cancer patients with special consideration for those who are frail. Antidepressant use in elderly patients should be titrated upward slowly (14).

Selective Serotonin Reuptake Inhibitors

SSRIs were introduced in the 1980s, replacing tricyclics as the antidepressants of choice in cancer patients because of fewer side effects. They are also the main long-term treatment of anxiety disorders, making them particularly useful in cancer patients, when depression and anxiety are often present simultaneously. Important drug interactions are inhibition of the P450 system and plasma binding. Common side effects, which usually dissipate, are headache, palpitations, nausea, inappropriate secretion of antidiuretic hormone, and sexual dysfunction due to an increase in serotonin levels (15).

Citalopram/escitalopram (Celexa®/Lexapro®, Forest) and sertraline (Zoloft®, Pfizer) have the lowest inhibition of the P450 system, and citalopram/escitalopram has the lowest binding to plasma protein. Fluoxetine (Prozac®, Dista) and paroxetine (Paxil®, GlaxoSmithKline) inhibit the P450 system to a greater extent and have higher plasma binding than the other SSRIs. Escitalopram often does not require a titration at the starting dose of 10 mg. Fluoxetine and its active metabolites have the longest half-life; paroxetine has no metabolites.

Serotonin and Norepinephrine Reuptake Inhibitors

Serotonin and norepinephrine reuptake inhibitors (SNRIs) have a dual action involving serotonin and norepinephrine. Currently, two SNRIs are available: venlafaxine (Effexor®, Wyeth) and duloxetine (Cymbalta®, Lilly). They are generally well tolerated and have a largely benign side effect profile, similar to the SSRIs. However, the inhibition of norepinephrine reuptake may cause nausea, palpitations, and hypertension. Venlafaxine comes in an extended-release form and has a unique action of mostly serotonin reuptake inhibition at lower doses and norepinephrine reuptake inhibition at higher doses of >150 mg. Venlafaxine must be titrated upwards slowly to prevent side effects (16). Duloxetine requires less titration than venlafaxine; the starting dose already shows inhibition of serotonin and norepinephrine. Both drugs have low P450 inhibition and moderate plasma binding (17). In addition to their usefulness in treating depression, venlafaxine and duloxetine are useful in treating neuropathic pain and hot flashes.

Table 3. Selected Medications for Treatment of Depression in Cancer Patients

	Starting Dose	Maintenance Dose	Comments
Selective serotonin reuptake inhibitors			
Citalopram (Celexa®, Forest)	10 mg qam	20–60 mg qam	Few drug interactions, low P450 inhibition and plasma binding
Escitalopram (Lexapro®, Forest)	10 mg qam	10–20 mg qam	Few drug interactions, low P450 inhibition and plasma binding
Fluoxetine (Prozac®, Dista)	10 mg qam	20–60 mg qam	Long half-life, more drug interactions through P450 inhibition
Paroxetine (Paxil®, Glaxo-SmithKline)	10 mg qam or qhs	20–60 mg qam or qhs	May be sedating, no active metabolites, P450 inhibition
Sertraline (Zoloft®, Pfizer)	25–50 mg qam	50–200 mg qam	Few drug interactions, low P450 inhibition
Serotonin/norepinephrine reuptake inhibitor			
Duloxetine (Cymbalta®, Lilly)	20–30 mg qam	30–60 mg qam	Activating, anxiety, nausea, few drug interactions
Venlafaxine (Effexor®, Wyeth)	37.5 mg qam	150–300 mg qam	Activating, requires titration, anxiety, nausea, few drug interactions (P450)
Norepinephrine antagonist/serotonin antagonist			
Mirtazapine (Remeron®, Organon)	7.5–30.0 mg qhs	15–45 mg qhs	Sedating, unusual dosing, weight gain, reduces nausea, appetite stimulant

Dopamine/norepinephrine reuptake inhibitor

Bupropion (Wellbutrin®, GlaxoSmithKline)	75–150 mg qam	150–450 mg qam	Activating, nausea, moderate P450 inhibition, requires titration

Stimulants/wakefulness-promoting agents

Methylphenidate (Ritalin®, GlaxoSmithKline)	2.5–5.0 mg qam	5–30 mg bid	Anxiety, agitation, nausea, cardiac side effects, requires titration
Dextroamphetamine (Adderall®, Shire US)	2.5–5.0 mg qam	5–20 mg bid	Anxiety, agitation, nausea, cardiac side effects, requires titration
Modafinil (Provigil®, Cephalon)	50–100 mg	100–400 mg	Activating, nausea, cardiac side effects, well tolerated

Norepinephrine Antagonists/Serotonin Antagonists

Mirtazapine (Remeron®, Organon) is a sedating dual-acting anti-depressant, which also has antiemetic properties and stimulates appetite, making it particularly useful in patients who are ano-rexic and debilitated. At lower doses, the sedating effect is greater; at higher doses of ≥30 mg, the sedating effect becomes less promi-nent and the antidepressant effect more pronounced. Sedation with bedtime dosing, increased appetite, and weight gain are side effects that are desirable in many patients with cancer. Interac-tions with the P450 system are minimal (18).

Dopamine and Norepinephrine Reuptake Inhibitor

Bupropion (Wellbutrin®, GlaxoSmithKline) is a dual-acting activat-ing antidepressant, which is useful in treating fatigue. It has the least sexual side effects and is tolerated well. It is also used for smoking ces-sation (Zyban®, GlaxoSmithKline) with good results. Side effects may include nausea, insomnia, anxiety, and palpitations. At higher doses, there is a risk of seizures; however, high doses are not common in cancer patients. Interaction with the P450 system is moderate. Immediate-, sustained-, and extended-release forms are available (16).

Tricyclics

Tricyclics are older antidepressants, which, because of their anticho-linergic, antiadrenergic, and antihistaminergic side effects, are less frequently used in patients with cancer. Common tricyclics are ami-triptyline (Elavil®, AstraZeneca), nortriptyline (Pamelor®, Mallinck-rodt), and desipramine (Norpramin®, Aventis). Side effects are orthostatic hypotension, sedation, blurred vision, and dry mouth at higher levels (19). The tricyclics are used largely for neuropathic pain and peripheral neuropathy in patients with cancer.

Stimulants and Wakefulness-Promoting Agents

Stimulants and wakefulness-promoting agents have a major advan-tage over antidepressants owing to their immediate onset of action and producing greater alertness, which diminishes fatigue, increases a sense of interest in activities, and counters the somnolence caused by opioids (20,21). Two stimulants used are dopaminergic: methylphen-idate (Ritalin®, GlaxoSmithKline) and dextroamphetamine (Adder-all®, Shire US). Side effects are anxiety, palpitations, restlessness, insomnia, and sometimes nausea; however, they are not common at low doses and can be avoided by starting at a low dose and titrating up to therapeutic effect. Hypertension and cardiac complications can occur, making it advisable to monitor cardiac function with a baseline electrocardiogram. When titrating to proper doses, the instant-release form is preferable. When maintenance level is reached, the extended-release forms may result in fewer side effects.

Modafinil (Provigil®, Cephalon) is a newer wakefulness-promoting agent, which acts on the hypocretin/orexin system in the lateral hypothalamus. It produces increased alertness, wakefulness, energy, and improved mood. It is better tolerated than the two stimulants mentioned earlier, but may also cause anxiety, restlessness, and insomnia. However, the half-life is short, and the dose can be reduced to prevent these side effects. In patients with hypertension, it should be used with caution (22,23).

Guidelines for Treatment

❖ Use antidepressants and stimulants in the treatment of depression.

Treatment of depression in the cancer setting depends on diagnosis, severity, and cause (24). Supportive psychological strategies and medication are useful. Suicidal ideation must be assessed and protective measures against suicide taken. Asking about suicidal intent does not increase the risk; moreover, the patient often feels relieved (25).

Adjustment disorders are often successfully treated with emotional support and counseling through a crisis period. Symptoms often remit with time and may not require psychopharmacologic intervention. However, severe adjustment disorders should be treated with an antidepressant, preferably an SSRI.

Major depressive disorder should be treated with psychological support and antidepressants. Psychostimulants are useful for fatigue and somnolence with fast onset of action. In the presence of neuropathic pain and hot flashes, SNRIs should be considered, and, when the primary symptom is insomnia, mirtazapine is preferable. Ongoing support, counseling, and psychotherapy are important. Medication given without support and careful monitoring is not recommended.

Mood disorder due to general medical condition, depressed type, can improve once the underlying cause is corrected. However, as this is

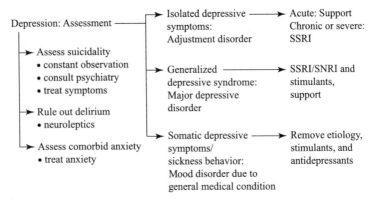

Figure 1
Depression algorithm. SNRI, serotonin and norepinephrine reuptake inhibitor; SSRI, selective serotonin reuptake inhibitor.

not often the case, an antidepressant is indicated, and the symptoms are treated as major depression. Paroxetine has been used prophylactically to prevent mood disorders related to interferon therapy (26). Psychostimulants, particularly modafinil, are useful for prominent fatigue.

Summary

❖ Adjustment disorder with depressed mood: support the patient and use antidepressants when severe or chronic.
❖ Major depressive disorder: provide psychological support and psychotherapy, start antidepressants, and consider stimulants for faster response.
❖ Mood disorder due to general medical condition, depressed: remove the underlying etiology and treat with SSRIs or stimulants, if necessary.
❖ Also see Figure 1.

Anxiety

Anxiety in cancer patients is extremely common, varying from fears and worries, which are normal, to symptoms of a formal anxiety disorder. *Adjustment disorder with anxious mood* is the most common, seen as situational or reactive anxiety, often in the presence of depressive symptoms. The common anxiety disorders in cancer are generalized anxiety disorder (GAD), panic disorder, specific phobia, and post-traumatic stress disorder (PTSD). Some symptoms of cancer (e.g., dyspnea), as well as a range of medications, can cause anxiety and are called *anxiety disorder due to general medical condition. Anxiety* is an emotional and physiologic response to a perceived threat with an increase in alertness, tension, and sympathetic nervous system response. Anxiety occurs at all stages of illness, and low levels of anxiety are regularly treated by the medical team with support and reassurance. Higher levels of anxiety may interfere with treatment compliance. Pain is a ubiquitous cause of anxiety, and the anxiety cannot be treated until the pain is controlled. Often the anxiety disappears once pain control has been achieved. Around one-third of patients experience significant anxiety with up to 50% reporting having it at some time (27–29).

Signs, Symptoms, and Diagnosis of Anxiety Disorders

Anxiety disorders (see Table 4 for DSM-IV criteria for anxiety disorders) common in cancer are diagnosed by the presence of several psychological and somatic signs and symptoms (2). Sudden onset of severe anxiety in patients with cancer may be the first sign of an impending serious medical event, particularly cardiovascular or respiratory. Thus, evaluation of anxiety must take this possibility into account first by a medical evaluation (30).

Psychological symptoms of anxiety are worry, irritability, and fright. Patients are hyperalert and hypervigilant, ruminate about fears, and may not be able to attend to their daily routine. Anxiety related to panic attacks comes on without a stimulus and with feelings of impending doom or death. Depersonalization and derealization are common. Patients with cancer who have had a severe prior trauma may re-experience the event with great anxiety and nightmares. Severe anxiety, which is overwhelming and intolerable, may be associated with suicidal ideation.

Table 4. DSM-IV Criteria for Selected Anxiety Disorders

Diagnosis	DSM-IV Criteria

Adjustment disorder
  With anxious mood
  With anxious/
    depressed mood
  Acute <6 mo
  Chronic >6 mo
	A. Development of emotional symptoms (nervousness, worry, jitteriness) in response to an identifiable stressor occurring within 3 mo
	B1. Marked distress in excess of expected level
	B2. Significant impairment in social or occupational functioning

Panic attack At least four symptoms develop abruptly and peak within 10 min	1. Palpitations 2. Sweating 3. Trembling or shaking 4. Shortness of breath or smothering 5. Feeling of choking 6. Chest pain or discomfort 7. Nausea or abdominal distress 8. Dizziness, lightheadedness, faintness 9. Depersonalization or derealization 10. Fear of losing control or going crazy 11. Fear of dying 12. Paresthesias 13. Chills or hot flashes
Specific phobias	A. Marked and persistent fear that is excessive or unreasonable regarding anticipation or presence of objects or situations B. Exposure to phobic stimuli almost invariably provokes an immediate anxiety response
Post-traumatic stress disorder	A. Experience or confrontation with a life-threatening event with a response of intense fear, helplessness, or horror B. Re-experience through intrusive recollections, recurrent dreams, reliving, and psychological and physiologic distress to symbols representing the traumatic event C. Avoidance of stimuli associated with the trauma D. Persistent symptoms of increased arousal, such as sleep, irritability, concentration, hypervigilance, startle response

Table 4. *Continued*

Diagnosis	DSM-IV Criteria
Generalized anxiety disorder	A. Excessive anxiety and worry occurring more days than not for at least 6 mo
	B. Difficulty in controlling worry
	C. Anxiety or worry associated with at least three of the following:
	1. Restlessness or feeling on edge
	2. Easily fatigued
	3. Difficulty concentrating or mind going blank
	4. Irritability
	5. Muscle tension
	6. Sleep disturbance
Anxiety disorder due to medical condition	A. Prominent anxiety or panic dominate the clinical picture
With generalized anxiety	B. Evidence for direct physiologic consequence of a general medical condition
With panic attacks	

DSM-IV, *Diagnostic and Statistical Manual of Mental Disorders*, 4th edition. Adapted from American Psychiatric Association. Diagnostic and Statistical Manual of Mental Disorders, 4th ed. Washington, DC: American Psychiatric Association, 1994.

Somatic signs of anxiety are as follows:

- ❖ Tachycardia
- ❖ Palpitations
- ❖ Elevated blood pressure
- ❖ Diaphoresis

Respiratory signs are as follows:

- ❖ Tightness in the chest
- ❖ Trouble breathing
- ❖ Tachypnea
- ❖ Shallow breathing, which leads to lightheadedness
- ❖ Dizziness

Gastrointestinal signs are as follows:

❖ Problems in swallowing
❖ Nausea
❖ Abdominal cramping
❖ Diarrhea

Adjustment Disorder with Anxious Mood

Hearing the diagnosis of cancer or hearing that it has progressed produces fears of death. Anxiety about the future and existential issues result in reactive anxiety that is called *adjustment disorder with anxious mood* in the DSM-IV. An adjustment disorder may resolve when the crisis is over, but it may become chronic and severe and require psychopharmacologic intervention along with counseling or psychotherapy.

Formal Anxiety Disorders: Panic Attacks, Specific Phobias, Generalized Anxiety Disorder, and Post-Traumatic Stress Disorder

Panic attacks and specific phobias are intermittent types of an anxiety disorder. *Panic attacks* are discrete episodes of intense fear or discomfort in the absence of real danger. There are three types:

❖ Unexpected (without precipitant)
❖ Situationally bound (anticipatory, e.g., claustrophobia)
❖ Situationally predisposed (anxiety prone)

Specific phobias are characterized by an excessive, unreasonable, and persistent fear of a specific object or situation. In cancer patients, fear of the sight of blood, a hospital room, chemotherapy, needles, and doctors are phobias that complicate care. A phobic response is seen in some cancer patients who develop anticipatory nausea and vomiting after several cycles of emetogenic chemotherapy. They begin to become nauseated en route to the hospital and before treatments that produce nausea and vomiting. A sense of anxiety can occur years later when the patient encounters a reminder of their treatment setting, such as seeing the nurse unexpectedly or experiencing a smell of the chemotherapy suite (31).

GAD is characterized by excessive anxiety and worry in everyday situations and particularly in relation to illness. Panic attacks may occur. Individuals with GAD may recognize that their anxiety and worry are irrational and excessive, but they are unable to control it.

PTSD is a term that was first used regarding Vietnam veterans, who were exposed to an extreme trauma with threat of death or injury. It now is used in relation to anxiety symptoms that result from frightening cancer treatments. Approximately 18%–20% of patients who have undergone bone marrow transplant show PTSD symptoms. Symptoms are nightmares, flashbacks, psychic numbing, reduced ability to experience emotion or pleasure, and feeling estranged (27).

Anxiety Disorder Due to Cancer and Treatment
Anxiety in the form of panic attacks or generalized anxiety can be caused by different physiologic factors (e.g., hypoxia, medication) and is classified as anxiety disorder due to general medical condition in the DSM-IV.

Etiology

The causes of anxiety are psychosocial, physical, and physiologic. Psychosocial factors that contribute are prior level of premorbid psychological functioning, immaturity, and lower resilience. Pain is the primary physical cause of anxiety, especially when it is uncontrolled or the patient fears it will return. A family history or past history of anxiety disorder predisposes the patient to its development during illness.

Medical factors causing anxiety are outlined in Table 5. Metabolic and endocrine problems and medications produce anxiety symptoms, which are classified as anxiety due to general medical condition. In the advanced stages of illness, anxiety disorders are very common. Symptoms of delirium (e.g., agitation, fear) may resemble an anxiety disorder, and it is important to differentiate between the two. Once the underlying cause is eliminated, anxiety disorders due to general medical condition may resolve, but antianxiety medication may be indicated.

Table 5.   Common Causes of Anxiety (Anxiety Due to General Medical Condition) in Cancer

Cancers	CNS neoplasms
	Carcinoid syndrome
Neurologic	Cerebrovascular disease
	Dementia/delirium
	Cerebral neoplasms
	Cerebral trauma
	CNS infections
Metabolic conditions	Vitamin deficiencies
	Hypoglycemia
Endocrine conditions	Adrenal abnormalities
	Thyroid abnormalities
	Parathyroid abnormalities
	Pituitary abnormalities
Systemic disorders	Hypoxia
	Cardiovascular disease
	Cardiac arrhythmias
	Pulmonary insufficiency
	Anemia
Medications/toxic conditions	Alcohol and drug withdrawal
	Akathisia related to antiemetics
	Caffeine and caffeine withdrawal
	Benzodiazepine withdrawal
	Amphetamines
	Sympathicomimetic agents
	Serotonergic agents
	Vasopressor agents
	Penicillin and sulfonamides
	Corticosteroids
Associated symptoms	Uncontrolled pain

CNS, central nervous system.

Management

Interventions are nonpharmacologic and pharmacologic. Non-pharmacologic interventions are psychologic support, psychotherapy, hypnosis, relaxation techniques, and meditation. Cognitive behavioral therapy is very helpful, but some patients prefer self-initiated interventions, such as relaxation techniques. Pharmacologic interventions are the use of benzodiazepines (BZDs), atypical neuroleptics, and antidepressants (Table 6) (32). Patients with severe anxiety benefit from an immediate effect. It is useful to start with a BZD or an atypical neuroleptic with a rapid action and combine it with an antidepressant with delayed onset of action, which is better for long-term maintenance therapy. Although antidepressants have a slow onset of action, they are the mainstay of treatment for anxiety disorder. Antidepressants take several weeks to reach therapeutic potential and usually require higher doses for anxiety than for depression (see Management section under Depression). Other agents, such as antihistamines and β-adrenergic antagonists, are helpful in milder forms of anxiety, but they often fail to relieve severe anxiety.

Benzodiazepines

BZDs act on the γ-aminobutyric acid-ergic system by binding to the BZD receptor and, through modulation, increase the chloride influx into the cell. All BZDs are anxiolytic. They provide fast relief and have few side effects, except for sedation, which may be desirable. Other advantages of BZDs are their antiemetic and muscle relaxing effects and availability for intravenous delivery (33). Interactions with other drugs are few (34). The major disadvantage is the development of physiologic dependence, which may make discontinuation difficult. A BZD should be tapered before stopping, and dosing over time may need to be increased owing to tolerance (35). In children, the elderly, and those with compromised brain function, BZDs may have a disinhibiting effect on behavior (36,37). Although several BZDs have a long half-life, it is better to use shorter-acting agents in doses given several times a day to monitor response and prevent sedation. The most useful BZDs are alprazolam (Xanax®, Pharmacia & Upjohn), clonazepam (Klonopin®, Roche Laboratories), diazepam (Valium®, Roche Products), and lorazepam (Ativan®, Baxter Anesthesia). Alprazolam is the shortest acting and may have the highest potential for physiologic dependence and development of withdrawal symp-

Table 6. Selected Medications for Treatment of Anxiety in Cancer Patients

	Starting Dose	Maintenance	Comments
Benzodiazepines			
Alprazolam (Xanax®, Pharmacia & Upjohn)	0.25–0.5 mg q4–8h	0.5–2.0 mg q4–8h	Short acting, less sedating
Clonazepam (Klonopin®, Roche Laboratories)	0.25–0.5 mg q6–8h	0.5–2.0 mg q6–8h	Medium half-life, sedating
Diazepam (Valium®, Roche Products)	2–5 mg q6–12h	5–10 mg q6–12h	Long acting, many metabolites, sedating
Lorazepam (Ativan®, Baxter Anesthesia)	0.5–1.0 mg q6–8h	0.5–2.0 mg q6–8h	Medium half-life, low plasma binding, no metabolites
Atypical neuroleptics (Serotonin/dopamine antagonists)			
Olanzapine (Zyprexa®, Lilly)	1.25–2.5 mg qhs or BID	2.5–5.0 mg qhs or BID	Sedating, metabolic syndrome
Quetiapine (Seroquel®, AstraZeneca)	12.5–25.0 mg qhs to TID	25–100 mg qhs to TID	Sedating, hypotensive, titration required
Risperidone (Risperdal®, Janssen)	0.25–1.0 mg qhs or BID	0.5–2.0 mg qhs or BID	Less sedating, hypotensive

Selective serotonin reuptake inhibitors

Citalopram (Celexa®, Forest)	10 mg qam	20–60 mg qam	Few drug interactions, low P450 inhibition and plasma binding
Escitalopram (Lexapro®, Forest)	10 mg qam	10–20 mg qam	Few drug interactions, low P450 inhibition and plasma binding
Fluoxetine (Prozac®, Dista)	10 mg qam	20–60 mg qam	Long half-life, more drug interactions through P450 inhibition
Paroxetine (Paxil®, GlaxoSmith-Kline)	10 mg qam or qhs	20–60 mg qam or qhs	May be sedating, no active metabolites, P450 inhibition
Sertraline (Zoloft®, Pfizer)	25–50 mg qam	50–200 mg qam	Few drug interactions, low P450 inhibition

Norepinephrine antagonist/serotonin antagonist

Mirtazapine (Remeron®, Organon)	7.5–30.0 mg qhs	15–45 mg qhs	Sedating, appetite stimulant, weight gain, reduces nausea

toms. Lorazepam and clonazepam have a midrange half-life and carry a lower risk of withdrawal symptoms. Lorazepam has the advantage of having no metabolites and is the preferable choice in the presence of compromised liver function. Diazepam has the longest half-life and has active metabolites. Active metabolites in the presence of compromised liver function increase the risk of oversedation.

Atypical Neuroleptics (Serotonin/Dopamine Antagonist)

Atypical neuroleptics (serotonin/dopamine antagonist), developed for the treatment of schizophrenia, have proven to be powerful anxiolytics. Their serotonergic, dopaminergic properties, and, in some atypical neuroleptics, antihistaminergic properties provide fast relief of anxiety. Some atypical neuroleptics are less sedating than BZDs and are useful adjuncts (38). At low doses, commonly used for anxiety, the side effect profile is benign (39). They also have a mild antidepressive effect and strong antiemetic effect.

Risperidone (Risperdal®, Janssen), olanzapine (Zyprexa®, Lilly), and quetiapine (Seroquel®, AstraZeneca) are the most useful as anxiolytics. Risperidone is the least sedating and is tolerated well.

Postural hypotension may occur owing to antiadrenergic effects and extrapyramidal side effects of dystonia and akathisia, and parkinsonian symptoms occur at higher doses.

Olanzapine and quetiapine have a low risk for extrapyramidal side effects. Olanzapine is sedating and is given at bedtime for insomnia. The major downside of olanzapine is the development of metabolic syndrome with weight gain, hyperglycemia, hypercholesterolemia, and hyperlipidemia, which limits its long-time use. Quetiapine has sedating and hypotensive properties and should be titrated starting at 25 mg. The half-life is short and may require doses two to three times a day. Its sedating quality makes it useful when given at bedtime for insomnia. Metabolic dysregulation usually does not occur.

Selective Serotonin Reuptake Inhibitors

SSRIs are best for long-term treatment of anxiety owing to their tolerability and efficacy. They are often combined with a BZD because of the SSRIs' slower onset of action. The doses are higher than in the treatment of depression and, thus, have more side effects. Norepinephrine antagonist/serotonin antagonist is more sedating than SSRIs. For a more detailed description of SSRIs and norepinephrine antagonist/serotonin antagonist, see the Selective

Serotonin Reuptake Inhibitors and Norepinephrine Antagonists/ Serotonin Antagonists sections under Depression.

❖ Use BZDs and atypical neuroleptics in the initial or temporary treatment of anxiety to produce an immediate effect.

❖ Use antidepressants for long-term treatment alone or in conjunction with BZDs or atypical neuroleptics.

Guidelines for Treatment

Anxiety in the cancer setting commonly occurs and should be treated depending on diagnosis, severity, and cause. Treatment of anxiety includes supportive strategies and medication.

Adjustment disorder with anxious mood is treated primarily with psychological support and counseling. Often symptoms remit with time and support, but severe adjustment disorder symptoms should be treated.

GAD and *panic disorder* are treated with psychotherapy and a combination of fast- and slow-onset medications: a BZD or atypical neuroleptics and an SSRI. *Specific phobias* are treated with psychotherapy, but anxiolytics may be necessary, especially when phobias interfere with treatment. *PTSD* is treated by cognitive behavioral psychotherapy and SSRIs, BZDs, or atypical neuroleptics depending on severity of symptoms.

Anxiety disorders due to general medical condition related to cancer or treatments are diminished when the underlying etiologic factor is eliminated (e.g., inhalers and corticosteroids for dyspnea). Often, they cannot be stopped, and BZDs and atypical neuroleptics are used, and, in chronic situations, an SSRI is the drug of choice.

Summary

❖ Adjustment disorder with anxious mood: support and use BZDs or atypical neuroleptics when severe or chronic.

❖ Anxiety disorders: psychological support and psychotherapy.
  ◆ GAD: BZDs and SSRIs
  ◆ Specific phobias: BZDs, when necessary
  ◆ Panic attacks: BZDs, atypical neuroleptics, and SSRIs
  ◆ PTSDs: BZDs, atypical neuroleptics, and SSRIs

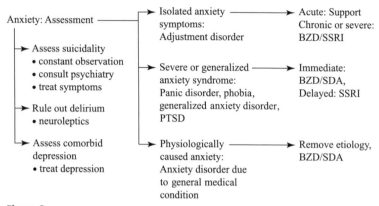

Figure 2
Anxiety algorithm. BZD, benzodiazepine; PTSD, post-traumatic stress disorder; SDA, serotonin/dopamine antagonist; SSRI, selective serotonin reuptake inhibitor.

- ❖ Anxiety disorder due to general medical condition: remove etiologic factor, when possible, and treat with BZDs, atypical neuroleptics, and SSRIs.
- ❖ Also see Figure 2.

Conclusion

Depression and anxiety are common emotions encountered by the oncologist. They are normal responses to cancer in the form of sadness, fears, and worries. However, the normal levels may increase to become a formal depressive and anxiety disorder. The oncologist must be able to recognize the symptoms that indicate that an anxiety or depressive disorder has developed that can interfere with cancer treatment. The chapter outlines signs, symptoms, and principles of management to assure that these symptoms are treated in the context of optimal supportive care.

References

1. Massie MJ. Prevalence of depression in patients with cancer. J Natl Cancer Inst Monogr 2004;32:57–71.

2. American Psychiatric Association. Diagnostic and Statistical Manual of Mental Disorders, 4th ed. Washington, DC: American Psychiatric Association, 1994.

3. Bottomley A. Depression in cancer patients: a literature review. Eur J Cancer Care (Engl) 1998;7:181–191.

4. Casey P. Adult adjustment disorder: a review of its current diagnostic status. J Psychiatr Pract 2001;7:32–40.

5. Winell J, Roth AJ. Depression in cancer patients. Oncology 2004; 18:1554–1560.

6. Pretorius E. Corticosteroids, depression and the role of serotonin. Rev Neurosci 2004;15:109–116.

7. Raison CL, Demetrashvili M, Capuron L, et al. Neuropsychiatric adverse effects of interferon-alpha: recognition and management. CNS Drugs 2005;19:105–123.

8. Leonard BE. The immune system, depression and the action of antidepressants. Prog Neuropsychopharmacol Biol Psychiatry 2001;25:767–780.

9. Yirmiya R, Weidenfeld J, Pollak Y, et al. Cytokines, "depression due to a general medical condition," and antidepressant drugs. Adv Exp Med Biol 1999;461:283–316.

10. Trask PC. Assessment of depression in cancer patients. J Natl Cancer Inst Monogr 2004;80–92.

11. Schwartz L, Lander M, Chochinov HM. Current management of depression in cancer patients. Oncology 2002;16:1102–1110.

12. Hemeryck A, Belpaire FM. Selective serotonin reuptake inhibitors and cytochrome P-450 mediated drug-drug interactions: an update. Curr Drug Metab 2002;3:13–37.

13. Frazer A, Benmansour S. Delayed pharmacological effects of antidepressants. Mol Psychiatry 2002;7(Suppl 1):S23–S28.

14. Joshi N, Breibart WS. Psychopharmacologic management during cancer treatment. Semin Clin Neuropsychiatry 2003;8:241–252.

15. Masand PS, Gupta S. Selective serotonin-reuptake inhibitors: an update. Harv Rev Psychiatry 1999;7:69–84.

16. Horst WD, Preskorn SH. Mechanisms of action and clinical characteristics of three atypical antidepressants: venlafaxine, nefazodone, bupropion. J Affect Disord 1998;51:237–254.

17. Dugan SE, Fuller MA. Duloxetine: a dual reuptake inhibitor. Ann Pharmacother 2004;38:2078–2085.

18. Nutt DJ. Tolerability and safety aspects of mirtazapine. Hum Psychopharmacol 2002;17(Suppl 1):S37–S41.

19. Masand PS. Tolerability and adherence issues in antidepressant therapy. Clin Ther 2003;25:2289–2304.

20. DeMarchi R, Bansal V, Hung A, et al. Review of awakening agents. Can J Neurol Sci 2005;32:4–17.
21. Morrow GR, Shelke AR, Roscoe JA, et al. Management of cancer-related fatigue. Cancer Invest 2005;23:229–239.
22. Robertson P Jr., Hellriegel ET. Clinical pharmacokinetic profile of modafinil. Clin Pharmacokinet 2003;42:123–137.
23. Wisor JP, Eriksson KS. Dopaminergic-adrenergic interactions in the wake promoting mechanism of modafinil. Neuroscience 2005;132:1027–1034.
24. Fisch M. Treatment of depression in cancer. J Natl Cancer Inst Monogr 2004;32:105–111.
25. Filiberti A, Ripamonti C. Suicide and suicidal thoughts in cancer patients. Tumori 2002;88:193–199.
26. Kraus MR, Schafer A, Scheurlen M. Paroxetine for the prevention of depression induced by interferon alfa. N Engl J Med 2001;345:375–376.
27. Bottomley A. Anxiety and the adult cancer patient. Eur J Cancer Care (Engl) 1998;7:217–224.
28. Stark D, Kiely M, Smith A, et al. Anxiety disorders in cancer patients: their nature, associations, and relation to quality of life. J Clin Oncol 2002;20:3137–3148.
29. Stark DP, House A. Anxiety in cancer patients. Br J Cancer 2000; 83:1261–1267.
30. Bowen RC. Differential diagnosis of anxiety disorders. Prog Neuropsychopharmacol Biol Psychiatry 1983;7:605–609.
31. Schag CA, Heinrich RL. Anxiety in medical situations: adult cancer patients. J Clin Psychol 1989;45:20–27.
32. Nutt DJ. Overview of diagnosis and drug treatments of anxiety disorders. CNS Spectr 2005;10:49–56.
33. Greenberg DB. Strategic use of benzodiazepines in cancer patients. Oncology 1991;5:83–88.
34. Tanaka E. Clinically significant pharmacokinetic drug interactions with benzodiazepines. J Clin Pharm Ther 1999;24:347–355.
35. Chouinard G. Issues in the clinical use of benzodiazepines: potency, withdrawal, and rebound. J Clin Psychiatry 2004;65(Suppl 5):7–12.
36. Stevens JC, Pollack MH. Benzodiazepines in clinical practice: consideration of their long-term use and alternative agents. J Clin Psychiatry 2005;66(Suppl 2):21–27.
37. Stiefel F, Berney A, Mazzocato C. Psychopharmacology in supportive care in cancer: a review for the clinician. I. Benzodiazepines. Support Care Cancer 1999;7:379–385.
38. Brawman-Mintzer O, Yonkers KA. New trends in the treatment of anxiety disorders. CNS Spectr 2004;9:19–27.
39. Ananth J, Parameswaran S, Gunatilake S. Side effects of atypical antipsychotic drugs. Curr Pharm Des 2004;10:2219–2229.

Index

Note: Page numbers followed by *t* indicate tables; those followed by *f* indicate figures.